STRATEGIC SKILLS FOR PUBLIC HEALTH PRACTICE SERIES

Systems and Strategic Thinking

For access to digital chapters,
visit the APHA Press bookstore (www.apha.org).

Strategic Skills for Public Health Practice Series
Series Editors: Michael Fraser, PhD, MS, and Brian C. Castrucci, DrPH

1. *Systems and Strategic Thinking*
2. *Policy Engagement*
3. *Resource Management and Finance*
4. *Community Engagement*
5. *Advancing Equity and Justice*
6. *Effective Communication*
7. *Change Management*
8. *Data-Informed Decision Making*
9. *Cross-Sectoral Partnerships*

STRATEGIC SKILLS FOR PUBLIC HEALTH PRACTICE SERIES

Systems and Strategic Thinking

Michael Fraser, PhD, MS

APHA PRESS
AN IMPRINT OF AMERICAN PUBLIC HEALTH ASSOCIATION

American Public Health Association
800 I Street, NW
Washington, DC 20001-3710
www.apha.org

Georges C. Benjamin, MD, MACP, Executive Director

Printed and bound in the United States of America
Book Production Editors: Maya Ribault, Keira McCarthy
Typesetting: The Charlesworth Group
Cover Design: Alan Giarcanella
Printing and Binding: Sheridan Books

Library of Congress Cataloging-in-Publication Data

Names: Fraser, Michael R., author. | American Public Health Association, issuing body.
Title: Systems and strategic thinking in public health / Michael R. Fraser.
Other titles: Strategic skills for public health practice series.
Description: Washington, DC : American Public Health Association, 2024. | Series: Strategic skills for public health practice series | Includes bibliographical references and index. | Summary: "At the core of the systems-and-strategic-thinking skill is an understanding of the need to approach problems and solutions from a big-picture perspective. The environments in which public health agencies operate are growing increasingly complex, thus requiring programs and interventions to be based in analyses of the systems to ensure the greatest impact"-- Provided by publisher.
Identifiers: LCCN 2024007117 (print) | LCCN 2024007118 (ebook) | ISBN 9780875533506 (paperback) | ISBN 9780875533513 (adobe pdf)
Subjects: MESH: Public Health Administration--methods | Systems Analysis | Strategic Planning
Classification: LCC RA425 (print) | LCC RA425 (ebook) | NLM WA 525 | DDC 362.1--dc23/eng/20240425
LC record available at https://lccn.loc.gov/2024007117
LC ebook record available at https://lccn.loc.gov/2024007118

To the many professionals who tirelessly champion the cause of public health and to the visionary thinkers who believe in the power of systems and strategic thinking to transform our world for the better.

Contents

Strategic Skills for Public Health Practice Series Introduction

Over the last 15 years, governmental public health professionals and partners nationwide have worked to define core competencies, essential services, and foundational capabilities of the public health.[1,2,3] Central to all these efforts is the public health workforce—the practitioners who work in local, state, territorial, tribal, and federal public health agencies to prevent disease and protect and promote the health of the public.

The governmental public health workforce is diverse and comprised of many technical specialties and professions. These professional identities have shaped public health practice and formed categories of work that comprise the organizational chart most governmental public health agencies utilize, such as maternal and child health, environmental health, epidemiology and surveillance, communicable disease control, administration and finance, school health, and several others.

These categories have served public health well by helping organize work and allowing for professionalization and leadership development within specific areas. Over 21 national professional associations represent categorical or function areas within state and territorial health departments alone, not to mention peer groups and affinity groups that are part of the Association of State and Territorial Health Officials and other allied organizations such as the National Association of County and City Health Officials, the Big Cities Health Coalition, CityMatCH (urban maternal and child health programs), the National Environmental Health Association, and others.

These specialty designations have also led to fragmentation within agencies at a time when government is attempting to align more nimbly to meet the needs of the jurisdictions they serve. Few public health professionals have formal training in the skills needed to successfully adapt their work to navigate these changes, especially the strategic skills needed to position their work to meet contemporary public health challenges that require inter- and intra-agency collaboration for success. For example, the pressures and challenges imposed on the public health ecosystem and its workers by the COVID-19 pandemic illustrate the urgency of preparing the public health workforce not just for technical challenges but also for strategic and adaptive challenges posed by novel health threats that require an "all of government" approach to resolve.

Several external forces in recent years, including the movement from Public Health 2.0 to Public Health 3.0 and the six-year-long, three-phased Public Health Workforce Interests and Needs Survey, have either advocated for or implied the need for complementing the workforce's existing discipline-specific expertise with developing a set of strategic skills.

In 2017, the de Beaumont Foundation spearheaded the development of the National Consortium for Public Health Workforce Development comprised of public health leaders from 34 national partner organizations representing a variety of disciplines and settings nationwide. The Consortium was established "to communicate the needs of the front-line public health worker to national partners and funders."[4]

By consensus, the Consortium identified the following nine "indispensable, high-performance skills applicable to the entire public health workforce regardless of specialty or discipline."[5]

- Systems and strategic thinking
- Change management
- Effective communication
- Data-informed decision making
- Community engagement
- Justice, equity, diversity, and inclusion
- Resource management and finance
- Policy engagement
- Cross-sectoral partnerships

These strategic skills are needed by specialty-specific, technical experts in order to realize the multisector, cross-cutting visionary leadership needed today. The Consortium's "call to action" paper asserted this challenge to public health educators: "While maintaining excellence in core scientific disciplines continues to be a priority, developers and deliverers of public health education and training need to act in new and different ways if the governmental public health workforce is to gain competency in the strategic skills needed throughout the entire public health workforce."[5]

Creating these "new and different ways" of building public health workforce competencies in the strategic skills should be a priority for academic programs, professional associations, and public health partners nationwide. This Strategic Skills Series presents a new way to expand the education and training of the public health workforce, equipping its members for multisector collaboration to create policies and programs intended to solve real problems.

To develop this series, we have recruited thought leaders and experts to serve as the authors of each volume. The consistent format applied to each book in the series is intended to facilitate the learner's absorption and retention of key concepts and applications. The practice-based objectives of each book in the series are described below:

- **Systems and strategic thinking:** Grasp patterns and relationships to understand systems contributing to public health problems and identify high-impact interventions.
- **Change management:** Scale programs in response to the changing environments and shape core elements that sustain programs in challenge and crisis.
- **Effective communication:** Convey resonant, compelling public health messages to broad audiences—the public, partners, and policymakers.
- **Data-informed decision making:** Leverage, synthesize, and analyze multiple sources of electronic data and use informatics to identify and act on health priorities, population impacts, evidence-based approaches, and health and cost-related outcomes.
- **Community engagement:** Describe the most effective methods of and the beneficial outcomes from engaging communities in promoting health and well-being. Promote the model of equitable distribution of decision-making power.
- **Justice, equity, diversity, and inclusion:** Understand and respond to the changing demographics of the US population and the public health workforce itself. Seek out, listen to, include, and promote underrepresented populations in reaching effective health solutions.
- **Resource management and finance:** Oversee recruitment, acquisition, and retention of the workforce and manage fiscal resources responsibly.
- **Policy engagement:** Address public health concerns and needs and engage effectively with local, state, and federal policymakers and partners.
- **Cross-sectoral partnerships:** Bring together two or more distinct fields (e.g., health care and transportation) for greater impact so that public health professionals can maintain long-term collaborations that combine a unique set of resources, experience, and knowledge to effectively address multifaceted issues (e.g., the social determinants of health).

As we aim to move public health forward to meet the challenges of contemporary practice, we are excited to edit each of these volumes. It is our fervent hope that each of the books in this series represents a significant brick in the foundation of developing your capacity to address today's urgencies as well as tomorrow's opportunities and challenges.

Michael Fraser, PhD, MS
Brian C. Castrucci, DrPH

REFERENCES

1. Public Health Foundation. Core competencies for public health professionals. 2014. Accessed January 22, 2021. http://www.phf.org/programs/corecompetencies/Pages/Core_Competencies_Domains.aspx
2. US Centers for Disease Control and Prevention. 10 essential public health services. 2020. Accessed August 30, 2024. https://www.cdc.gov/public-health-gateway/php/about/index.html

3. Public Health National Center for Innovation. Foundational public health services. 2018. Accessed August 30, 2024. https://phaboard.org/wp-content/uploads/FPHS-Factsheet-2022.pdf
4. de Beaumont Foundation. Building skills for a more strategic public health workforce: a call to action. 2019. Accessed September 26, 2022. https://debeaumont.org/wp-content/uploads/2019/04/Building- Skills-for-a-More-Strategic-Public-Health-Workforce.pdf
5. de Beaumont Foundation. Building skills for a more strategic public health workforce: a call to action. July 18, 2017. Accessed January 22, 2021. https://www.debeaumont.org/news/2017/building-skills-for-a-more-strategic-health-workforce-a-call-to-action

Acknowledgments

Creating a brief primer on a massive topic such as systems and strategic thinking in public health was a Herculean task made easier by the contributions of many. Many thanks to Keri Vareen, who supported efforts to obtain permissions to reproduce images and diagrams in this volume. Thanks to colleague and friend Dr. Brian C. Castrucci for his support in the conceptualization of the strategic skills in the first place, and for his encouragement to author this volume. Many thanks to Dan Doody and Maya Ribault for their editorial support through the development and final publication process. Finally, many thanks to Zarnaaz Bashir, Dr. John Davidoff, and Jane Branscomb for their inspiration to think strategically and for sharing their systems and strategic thinking expertise with me. I am truly grateful.

Introduction: A Tale of Two Systems

For years, public health professionals have been working to reduce the rate of infant mortality in the United States, and have had some success: the rate in 2020 was at a historic low of 5.4 per 1,000 births.[1] However, persistent and pervasive racial inequities have led to a gap between white and nonwhite infant death rates, with Black and American Indian/Alaska Native rates in some states being two to three times higher than whites. In a 2023 study on infant deaths published in the journal *Pediatrics*, researchers reported that even with a declining overall rate of infant death, sudden unexpected deaths among infants increased between 2019 and 2020, with the largest spike in sudden unexplained infant death syndrome (SUIDS) among Black infants.[2]

Infant mortality has been a core measure of the country's health for decades. The US has spent billions of public health and health care dollars to improve access to and quality of maternal and infant health services. Entire program areas within local, state, tribal, territorial, and federal public health agencies focus on maternal and child health, with core investments in maternal and infant death reviews, early childhood home visitation programs, and programs to prevent infant death through parental education on safer sleep practices. Hundreds of nonprofit groups, medical professional associations, and health care organizations have invested their resources in closing the racial gap and reducing infant deaths, including SUIDS, for years. How can this gap remain?

In a commentary responding to the 2023 study from the journal *Pediatrics*, Carlin and colleagues stated that the persistent gap in infant mortality rates by race and the spike in sudden deaths among Black infants "reflect our societal failures,"[3(p2)] noting the following:

> The United States has one of the highest SUID rates for all middle- and high-income countries… and the findings regarding increasing disparities sound the alarm about the need for interventions that look beyond individual counseling and toward community- and society-level solutions. All infants deserve a better start in life than we in the United States are providing to them now.[3(p2)]

Persistent. Long-standing. The need to move from individual level toward community and societal level solutions. These terms and phrases are important indicators of the need to think about the system that generates these results. A constellation of interconnected factors, not just one cause, produces the racial gap in SUIDS outcomes. The need to look holistically at a problem to understand it, and then attempt solve it, requires systems and strategic thinking.

The infant mortality/SUIDS system, defined here as the set of interrelated parts that produces the current rate of infant deaths and deaths specific to SUIDS, is a complex network of individuals, families, neighborhoods, public health agencies, health care organizations, clinical resources, neighborhood assets, educational organizations, housing and employment services, and the relationships between them. To make a significant reduction in the SUIDS rate, we must look at these components and their relationships, and the outcomes and inequities that this system yields. That analysis, a systems approach, can identify where there are points for improvement that could lead to better infant health outcomes.

Importantly, it is critical to note that the increased rate for SUIDS among Black infants may be unintentional, but it is not accidental or due to chance.[2] A system produces that result whether it is intended or not. The good news? Systems can be changed. The bad news? It is overwhelming to think about the system improvements needed to make such changes.

Take another pressing health threat: global climate change. We have known for years that our planet's surface is getting warmer due to many factors, including greenhouse gas emissions from industrial and consumer burning of fossil fuels. As a result, a warming ocean melts more sea ice. Entire island nations in the Pacific region now face the existential challenge of migrating from their atoll and island homelands to higher ground in other parts of the world.[4] These migrations are largely due to the catastrophic impact of flooding from stronger and stronger typhoons, higher and higher King Tides, and other significant weather events. Regions around the globe are experiencing major temperature extremes and the resultant wildfires, drought, and stronger tornadoes. Increasing temperatures create the conditions for disease vectors and viruses to move to previously unexposed regions of the globe as warming climates make new areas more hospitable to them, increasing disease risks.

In response to a warming climate, national and international initiatives have focused on several contributors to global warming, including reducing greenhouse emissions, by creating more efficient cars and greening factories to reduce the use of fossil fuels. Certainly, reducing fossil fuels will help. However, a recent study found that over 30 different feedback loops contribute to global climate change.[5,6] Feedback loops push and pull each other and collectively impact seemingly unrelated parts of the climate system, like wildfire risk and childhood asthma or melting Alaskan tundra and an increase in tick-borne infectious diseases. To achieve the goal of slowing climate change, interventions must comprehensively understand all the interrelated components of the climate and health system and examine their interplay to generate effective interventions.

Big picture. Interrelatedness of parts. Comprehensive. Feedback loops. Again, these terms and phrases are key indicators of the need to use the systems and strategic thinking skill to address the complexity of many major issues in contemporary public health practice. Infant death and the impact of climate change on health are just two of the many examples of how systems and strategic thinking can be applied in public health. The purpose of this primer is to introduce you to the strategic skill of systems and strategic thinking and provide you with some tips and tools to start applying this skill to your work in public health practice.

WHAT ARE THE STRATEGIC SKILLS?

Research on the public health workforce and feedback from meetings of public health leaders working at the local, state, and federal levels has emphasized the need for public health practitioners to complement their technical proficiency in specific domains of public health practice with strategic skills that crosscut disciplines and programmatic categories.[7] The strategic skills are not specific to any specific public health specialty or focus area such as maternal and child health, epidemiology, or chronic disease prevention. Rather, the strategic skills are broad competencies needed by public health practitioners in any area of public health practice to successfully perform public health activities.

Employers want and need employees who can think systematically and strategically. In the organization I lead, the Association of State and Territorial Health Officials (ASTHO), I often push our staff to think more strategically. With all the tactical work of grants and planning, and the seemingly endless work of program administration and project management, it is sometimes difficult for staff to remember why they are doing their work in the first place. It takes effort to dedicate time to thinking about how all the pieces fit together across a large organization and across the work of stakeholders in sectors adjacent to public health. Systems and strategic thinking, however, requires just such an approach.

Recently, an exasperated staff member said to me, "I know you want us to think more strategically, but you need to tell us how! We can't read your mind." Fair point. To my team, and the many others who want some help in developing their strategic and systems thinking competency, this primer is for you. It includes specific examples of prompts and approaches that anyone can use to think systematically and strategically. It makes the case for why systems and strategic thinking needs to be integrated into public health planning and decision-making at all levels of a public health organization. The central premise of this primer is that for public health professionals to truly promote and protect the health of their communities, they must apply systems and strategic thinking to their community's most pressing and difficult-to-solve public health challenges.

WHY SYSTEMS AND STRATEGIC THINKING MATTERS

If there was ever a time for public health professionals to develop and enhance their systems and strategic thinking competency, it is now. The lasting effects of the COVID pandemic on public health agency operations, the politicization of public health measures such as mask mandates and vaccination requirements, and the increasingly close connections between public health agencies, healthcare, and related sectors require public health leaders to engage in discussions about their agencies' strategic positioning and the systems in which their agencies operate.

Creating meaningful improvements to some of our most vexing public health challenges involves looking closely at the systems and structures that produce inequities and poor health outcomes. During the COVID pandemic, we all observed in real time that COVID infections and severe illness decreased when we intervened at multiple leverage points in the COVID response system. These included comprehensive policies and programmatic decisions such as making vaccines available without any co-pay, expanding vaccination sites, and making them accessible to communities hardest hit by the pandemic. They also included promoting the deployment of community health workers to share health information, linking people to care by addressing social needs such as grocery delivery that made isolation and quarantine easier, and policy changes such as expanding paid sick leave. In short, a systems approach to COVID required quickly mapping out all the parts of the COVID response system, examining the interplay of public health and many other sectors, and leveraging interventions where we could have the most impact on preventing infections.

At the core of the systems and strategic thinking skill is an understanding of the need to approach problems and solutions from a broad, big-picture perspective. The National Consortium for Public Health Workforce Development (the Consortium) uses this definition of systems and strategic thinking:

> A holistic and dynamic understanding of interrelated complex structures—such as public health and health care—as well as the ability to recognize those systems' influences at multiple levels and use those insights to align resources to achieve goals. It involves designing interventions that help people see the overall structures, patterns, and cycles in systems and allows for the identification of solutions that simultaneously leverage improvement throughout the system.[7(p21)]

The Consortium uses one term to combine both systems thinking and strategic thinking. These two terms, systems thinking and strategic thinking, are often separately addressed in the organizational behavior and management literature. Combining the two into the one strategic skill of systems and strategic thinking allows us to focus on the core attribute of both systems and strategy: a holistic view that recognizes the interdependencies and interconnectedness of the elements that produce particular results and potential futures. The systems and strategic thinking skill is desired by many public health professionals. The Public Health Workforce Interests and Needs Survey (PH WINS) conducted in 2021 found that 47% of all public health workers identified systems and strategic thinking as a training need, second only to budget and financial management.[8] The need for systems and strategic skill training was expressed as a particular need by supervisors, mangers, and executives (54%) compared with nonsupervisory staff (44%).[8] This primer introduces foundational systems and strategic thinking concepts that public health professionals can use to get started. It also suggests resources for further study to increase your knowledge in this skill area through additional trainings and recommendations for further study.

The systems and strategic thinking skill is important because the environments in which public health agencies operate are growing increasingly complex and public health professionals are increasingly aware of the social, political, and economic factors that influence health outcomes. This complexity means that public health programs and interventions, including partnerships that promote health, should be based in analyses of the systems in which public health work is taking place to have the most impact. Band-aid approaches and siloed public health interventions are insufficient to produce the system changes needed to sustain the long-term health improvement to which we all aspire. Just as military planners adjusted the way they trained and organized to fight in an increasingly volatile, uncertain, complex, and ambiguous environment of increasing global terrorism, public health practitioners have had to adjust the way they respond to emerging and persistent health threats using systems and strategic thinking.

At the enterprise level, many public health agencies are collections of disparate programs, usually organized by common disease states or topical areas such as chronic disease prevention, infectious disease control, or maternal and family health. These programmatic verticals, often referred to as silos, are helpful ways to consolidate similar work and related funding and program management activities. A focus on only verticals, however, can inhibit important crosscutting or horizontal work across functional areas that is required to think in systems and think strategically.

For example, health equity work in public health agencies is often organized as an "office of" or "division for" health equity where an agency's equity work is centralized. This means that teams have to reach across program silos (go horizontal) to connect with other agency programs and functional areas (the verticals) to link to and collaborate with others doing equity work. The work of systems and strategic thinking requires this horizontal perspective, working across an organization to identify resources and initiatives that advance shared strategic goals.

At ASTHO, our priority is to meet the strategic goals identified by our Board of Directors as expressed in our strategic plan priorities and related objectives. ASTHO staff use strategic thinking to align the priorities our board has set with the resources obtained to do that work. Similarly, in health departments, strategic thinking is the process that organizational managers and leaders can use to share overarching goals with their teams, elected officials, and policymakers. Strategic thinking promotes the alignment of various agency functions and activities toward common goals and priorities.

Systems and strategic thinking in public health therefore matters a great deal if an organization expects to improve the health of their community. For example, if childhood obesity prevention is a priority, agency staff will have to move beyond a vertical nutrition program and connect with partners supporting physical activity programs. This means connecting with the work of schools, environment and recreation partners, food systems partners, and parent- and child-serving groups in their community. Teams can use systems and strategic thinking to position and align their work within a program area. They can also use it to connect their work with efforts across the organization to meet shared agency goals and contribute to the goals and priorities of external partners.

REFERENCES

1. Ely DM, Driscoll AK. Infant mortality in the United States, 2020: Data from the period linked birth/infant death file. *Natl Vital Stat Rep*. 2022;71(5):1–18. doi:10.15620/cdc:120700
2. Shapiro-Mendoza CK, Woodworth KR, Cottengim CR, et al. Sudden unexpected infant deaths: 2015–2020. *Pediatrics*. 2023;151(4):e2022058820. doi:10.1542/peds.2022-058820
3. Carlin RF, Hauck FR, Moon RY. Increasing disparities in sudden unexpected infant deaths reflect societal failures. *Pediatrics*. 2023;151(4):ee2022060798. doi:10.1542/peds.2022-060798
4. Miller M. A sinking nation is offered an escape route. But there's a catch. *The Washington Post*. December 26, 2023. Accessed January 2, 2024. https://www.washingtonpost.com/world/2023/12/26/australia-tuvalu-deal-climate-change-pacific
5. Ripple WJ, Wolf C, Lenton TM, et al. Many risky feedback loops amplify the need for climate action. *One Earth*. 2023;6(2):86–91. doi:10.1016/j.oneear.2023.01.004
6. Paddison L. Nearly 30 dangerous feedback loops could permanently shift the Earth's climate, scientists say. *CNN*. February 17, 2023. Accessed January 2, 2024. https://www.cnn.com/2023/02/17/world/climate-feedback-loops-tipping-points-arctic-ice-intl
7. de Beaumont Foundation. Adapting and aligning public health strategic skills. 2021. Accessed January 2, 2024. https://debeaumont.org/wp-content/uploads/2021/04/Adapting-and-Aligning-Public-Health-Strategic-Skills.pdf
8. de Beaumont Foundation and the Association of State and Territorial Health Officials (ASTHO). PH Wins 2021 National Dashboard. July 31, 2023. Accessed January 2, 2024. https://www.phwins.org/national

1

What Is Systems Thinking?

Systems thinking is an approach to problem-solving and decision-making that emphasizes the interconnectedness and interactions of different parts of a system. The important insight of systems thinking is the idea that our work plays out in a world where everything is connected, and that changing one part of the system can have impact on another part of the system. It encourages us to look beyond simple cause-and-effect relationships and consider the many factors that produce a given situation or outcome.

The first time I learned about systems thinking, my instructor used the example of automobile traffic and road congestion. Think about a common approach to solving traffic problems and congestion: build more roads. It does seem obvious that building more roads, or widening the ones that are overcrowded, is a simple and commonsense approach to helping ease traffic. But have you ever noticed what happens when new roads are built, or existing roads are widened? While there may be a temporary easing of traffic, they ultimately get crowded again as more people use the roads. This then leads to a repeat of the original problem, only worse because there is more traffic, not less. What is going on here?

To start, we have to understand the transportation system producing the outcome we are seeking to change. What are its parts, such as roads and cars, but also rideshare, public transit, dedicated bicycle lanes, and walkable and safe sidewalks, that offer alternatives to cars? What are the attitudes and beliefs about the system and its parts? In the US, there is an ethos that promotes car ownership and that has led to the proliferation of the automobile. It has also led to a lack of investment in alternatives to cars, such as reliable public transportation, in many areas. The costs of parking and driving are also parts of the system. Safety concerns influence decisions to share transit, or to brave traffic by riding one's bike. Lack of sidewalks or poorly placed crosswalks may limit pedestrian options and push people to drive instead, contributing to traffic volume.

The system also includes attitudes and mindsets about socioeconomic status and the prestige of driving one's own car, as well as stereotypes and prejudices about who uses public transportation. In short, this brief transportation system analysis suggests that the traffic problem we seek to change has to do with a lot more than cars and roads. Taking a systems thinking approach to the transportation system includes examining all the transportation options in a community, and the beliefs about and interactions between components in the system. The systems thinker then looks at these relationships and identifies points of intervention, called leverage points, in systems. A sustainable solution to increasing traffic may not include the seemingly commonsense intervention of building more roads. Instead, a solution might include supporting a number of interventions like building more sidewalks, addressing concerns about the safety of public transportation, and changing mindsets about the necessity of car ownership, to name just a few.

Preventing opioid overdose deaths is also a complex problem. By not taking a systems and strategic thinking perspective, however, many well-intentioned interventions to prevent overdose deaths may have unintentionally made the problem worse. It seems logical that reducing the supply of opioids in a community by using a prescription drug monitoring program (PDMP) to monitor opioid prescriptions and requiring prescribers to follow consensus guidelines when prescribing opioids would reduce the volume of opioids in a community and reduce the rate of opioid overdose. In some communities, PDMPs and opioid prescribing guidelines have had that effect. But in other communities with the same interventions (PDMP use and prescribing guidelines), overdose deaths from opioids continue to rise. What is going on?

Most likely, these system changes reducing the licit opioid supply may have had the consequence of pushing some individuals to seek out and use illicit opioids, like heroin, instead. The increased supply of the extremely dangerous drug fentanyl in the illicit drug supply has made heroin use even more deadly. Limiting opioid prescribing may have inadvertently caused more people to seek illicit opioids, which increased their risk of overdose death. In any system, a change to one part impacts the dynamics of the other parts. Without taking a systems approach, well-intended changes can lead to unintended consequences and a worsening of the system's results.

In short, single cause–effect solutions like building more roads or requiring opioid prescriptions to be entered into a database may be impactful, especially in the short term. But these solutions only address parts of a much larger system-level problem that ultimately may return over time. In the overdose example, mapping out the opioid overdose system to look at the entirety of the system and the components that work to prevent overdoses requires identifying points of intervention beyond a PDMP. Other leverage points such as efforts to interrupt the fentanyl supply and public health efforts to promote the primary prevention of addiction would lead to more comprehensive systems change and more lasting health improvements.

Donella Meadows, a pioneer in the field of systems thinking who is referred to frequently in this volume, uses this definition of a system: a system is "an interconnected set of elements that is coherently organized in a way that achieves something."[1(p11)] Her definition emphasizes that a system is more than just collections of things. They are parts coherently organized and interconnected to achieve a particular purpose or goal. And while it is important to think about systems as a set of connected parts, it is also important to remember that a system's connections are ultimately maintained through relationships between people. Public health leadership scholar Louis Rowitz reminds us that systems are in fact more than just the sum of their parts, they include the relationships between people that enable the system to function.[2] These relationships include mindsets and behaviors that influence system outcomes.

In their chapter "Systems Thinking for Public Health Professionals," Branscomb and colleagues refer to a systems "mindset," or a way of thinking that emphasizes connections, relationships, and patterns:

> [A] system is a set of interacting components and the structures governing how they interact to produce certain results over time. Components can be all sorts of things, both tangible and abstract, such as people, buildings, knowledge, technology, mindsets, and more. Structures, too, can be tangible or abstract, and include physical arrangements, spatial relationships, stated or implicit rules, policies, and norms. Systems thinking starts with a systems mindset: the recognition that the outcome trend we get is the result of a system in operation. The skill of systems thinking is that of accurately discerning and understanding the system driving certain results.[3(pp39–40)]

In the context of this public health–focused primer, we will define a system as the set of components and structures and the relationships and connections between people in communities that produce specific health outcomes and promote or prevent the conditions necessary for health and well-being. A public health systems thinker uses the tools of systems thinking to identify how the system produces such outcomes and leverage opportunities for intervention and improvement.

USING SYSTEMS THINKING IN PUBLIC HEALTH

There are many ways that public health professionals can use systems thinking in their work. Public health professionals' focus on health equity, anti-racism, and addressing the social determinants of health requires a systems approach because these are issues that cannot be addressed by a single program or policy intervention. As stated, the interplay of many components creates the various systems within which public health is practiced. Four characteristics of public health describe why systems thinking is applicable to public health practice: (1) public health problems are complex, (2) solutions to public health problems require many different sectors working together, (3) public health focuses on sustainability, and (4) public health is ripe for innovation.

Public Health Problems Are Complex

Most of the public health problems we face are complex and involve multiple factors that interact with each other in nonlinear ways across many different sectors. Systems thinking provides a framework for examining complex systems and identifying the underlying causes of specific outcomes.

Public Health Problems Require the Engagement of Many Sectors

Systems thinking takes the view that everything in the world is interconnected. Public health practice is often referred to as a team sport because of its interconnectedness to other sectors and stakeholders and the need to span organizational boundaries to reach public health goals. Systems thinking tools, especially causal loop diagrams, can be used to help illustrate how different parts of a system are linked together and how the parts interact and connect across sectors to produce specific outcomes.

Public Health Focuses on Sustainability

As public health practitioners face environmental and social challenges such as the health effects of climate change, poverty, and inequality, systems thinking can help practitioners design more sustainable solutions. By taking a holistic view of these issues and considering the entire system, public health professionals can identify leverage points where small changes may have a big impact and lead to more efficient use of resources and more lasting impact.

Public Health Is Ripe for Innovation

In the wake of the global COVID pandemic and in response to the challenges and opportunities it presented to the public health system, public health leaders are now considering new ways to protect and promote health and prevent disease. Systems thinking can help practitioners identify opportunities for innovation and change in these agencies by looking at a problem from multiple angles and considering different perspectives. These different perspectives can help public health professionals innovate new and creative solutions that might not have been apparent before COVID or when taking a narrow view of a problem.

PUBLIC HEALTH AND SYSTEMS THINKING

Once you decide to take a systems thinking approach to a public health issue, it is important to ask a variety of questions to gain a full understanding of the system being analyzed. Here are some of the questions you can use to develop your systems thinking competency, based on work by systems thinking experts Donella Meadows and Peter Senge[1,4]:

1. What are the system's boundaries and how are they defined? This question helps to identify the scope of the system being studied and how it interacts with other parts of the environment or its context impacting the issue.
2. What are the key components of the system and how do they interact with each other? Identifying the components of the system and how they are connected helps reveal the underlying structure and dynamics of the system.

3. What are the feedback loops within the system and how do they impact system behavior? Feedback loops can either reinforce, diminish, or balance system behavior, and understanding these dynamics is essential to systems change.
4. How does the system evolve over time and what are the key factors that drive system change? Understanding the evolution of the system over time, as well as its future trajectory, is essential to systems thinking.
5. What are the system's goals, and from what different perspectives can these goals be assessed? Identifying the goals of the system and how these goals are accomplished can reveal important insights into system behavior and the relationships between the parts of the system.

These questions and your answers to them will push you to consider the entirety of a system rather than just a part of it. Thinking in systems can be novel to many public health professionals used to working in a specific specialty area or on a narrow topic. Formal scientific and technical training in public health often emphasizes reductionist approaches to understanding public health problems. Reductionism breaks down complex systems or problems into their individual components and focuses on understanding and analyzing each component in isolation.

In public health, reductionist thinking may involve looking at a specific disease or health issue and studying it in detail, often through the lens of biology, chemistry, or epidemiology. This approach posits that by understanding the individual parts, you gain insights into the whole system. However, looking at individual parts may also mean missing larger connections and links between components that might seem inconsequential at the micro level but have bigger implications for the system. Public health analyses understandably require reducing complicated problems to as finite a set of factors as possible and then, often using statistical analysis, looking for relationships between the factors such as cause and effect.

Reductionism has value: it can provide detailed insights into the specific components of a system. It also allows for in-depth understanding of certain aspects of public health. However, reductionism can oversimplify complex problems and may miss the interconnected factors that are related to a system's outcomes. In practice, public health work requires a balance between reductionist and systems thinking approaches. Incorporating systems thinking is crucial for addressing complex, multifaceted health challenges because it uncovers the root causes and interconnections between various factors, making it possible to develop more comprehensive and effective interventions.

SYSTEMS THINKING TOOLS

This section presents several systems thinking tools, including feedback loops, cause-and-effect diagrams, stock-and-flow diagrams, and behavior-over-time graphs. These tools are helpful in getting you started on your systems thinking journey.

A Process for Making a System Visible

To help define a system, it is important to ask a set of questions. These include the following: What is the purpose of the system? What are its parts, and how are they connected? What stakeholders are part of the system? What are the boundaries of the system? What is characteristic of the system and its outcomes? Who benefits from system outcomes? Who is disadvantaged by them? Why?

Define the System's Purpose

Start by clearly defining the public health issue you want to address and what you are trying to achieve. This will set the context and parameters for your system boundaries. Questions that help identify the system's purpose include: What is the stated purpose of the system? What are its outcomes, including intended and unintended results? What are the consequences of the system? Answers to these questions will help you articulate the purpose of the system and get started on defining its components and their relationships.

Identify Key Components and Stakeholders

After assessing the system's purpose, explore the main components, stakeholders, and relationships relevant to the system. To broaden your scope, be sure to not only use sources familiar to you but also published literature on the topic, public health reports, commentaries, and/or expert opinions. The World Health Organization's (WHO) Health Systems Building Blocks framework is used to examine global health systems and may help you define and examine specific parts of a system.[5] The six building blocks in the framework include the following: (1) financing, (2) health workforce, (3) information systems, (4) medical products, vaccines, and technologies, (5) leadership and governance, and (6) service delivery. For each of these building blocks, ask these questions: What are the components and relationships in this part of the system? What stakeholders are involved? What connections link the system's parts? You can then broaden your analysis to other sectors, including adjacent sectors in the public health system. You can also develop your own set of building blocks to complement those developed by WHO.

Analyze Interconnections and Relationships

Next, explore how the components you identified interact with each other within the broader system. Use feedback loops and causal relationships to diagram these interactions (more on these later). Once the components of the system are identified, analyze how they relate to each other. This involves exploring how input and output loops relate to different components of the system. Diagramming these relationships can help make the connections between them visible and is an important step in systems thinking.

Set System Boundaries

Define the boundaries of the system based on the components and relationships identified. Be aware that system boundaries may expand as you further your analysis. Part of setting boundaries may include consulting with community groups and other public health or community stakeholders to revise and adjust your understanding of the system's boundaries and how components are related to other systems.

Involve Stakeholders

Systems thinking is not just an individual practice but requires the participation of many different groups. Engage others to fully define the boundaries and components of a system. Stakeholders, subject matter experts, and those with lived experience can bring diverse perspectives to your analysis and help define system purpose, components, connections, and boundaries.

Feedback Loops and Causal Loop Diagrams

Feedback loops and causal loop diagrams are essential tools used in systems thinking. A feedback loop occurs when the output of a system is fed back into the system as an input, creating a loop of information or action.[1,2] There are two main types of feedback loops: balancing and reinforcing. A reinforcing feedback loop has an amplifying effect in which an action produces more of, or less of, the same action, leading to an increase or decrease over time. A balancing feedback loop can increase or decrease the effects of a change back to a desired state. Feedback loops can create stability (balancing) or instability (reinforcing) within a system, depending on their nature and strength.[1]

Reinforcing Feedback Loops

Reinforcing feedback loops in public health can amplify the impact of health-related factors and lead to either positive or negative outcomes in a system. Figure 1-1 shows the birth rate and population size feedback loop: as births increase, the population increases, and as the population increases, the birth rate increases. Reinforcing loops lead to instability or change in a system, including exponential growth or decline. Some examples of reinforcing feedback loops in public health include the following:

1. Infectious disease spread: When a contagious disease spreads rapidly, it can create a positive feedback loop. As more people become infected, the likelihood of transmitting the disease to others increases, leading to an increase in infections.
2. Health education: Effective health education programs can create a positive feedback loop. When individuals receive education on healthy behaviors, they are more likely

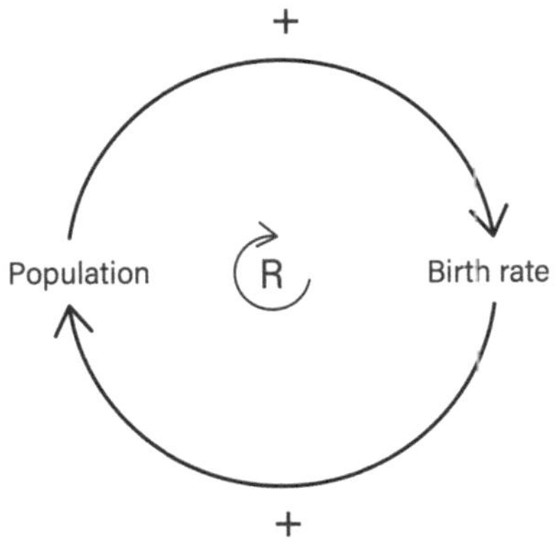

Note: A "+" or a "−" in the loop diagram indicates the nature of the action (increase or decrease). An "R" with an arrow around it is the symbol used to denote a reinforcing loop. A "B" with an arrow around it is the symbol used to denote a balancing loop.

Figure 1-1. Positive Reinforcing Feedback Loop Examples: Birth Rate and Population Size

to adopt these behaviors. As more people adopt healthy habits, the overall health of the community improves, creating a virtuous cycle of better health.

3. Smoking cessation: Programs that help people quit smoking can lead to positive feedback loops. When individuals successfully quit smoking, they often become advocates for cessation, encouraging others to do the same. This can result in more people quitting and, in turn, advocating for more smoking cessation resources.
4. Improving access to maternal health services: Improvements in maternal health can create a positive feedback loop. When women have access to better prenatal care, safe deliveries, and postpartum support, both maternal and infant health outcomes improve. Healthier mothers are more likely to have healthy children, reinforcing better maternal and child health.
5. Immunization campaigns: Immunization campaigns create negative feedback loops. As more people in a community get vaccinated against infectious diseases, the prevalence of the disease decreases. This, in turn, reduces the chances of the disease spreading further, contributing to overall community immunity and reduced disease incidence.
6. Anti-smoking regulations: Policies and regulations aimed at reducing tobacco use create negative feedback loops. These measures discourage smoking and, over time, lead to reduced smoking rates and associated health risks.
7. Contact tracing and disease investigation: Effective contact tracing during disease outbreaks creates negative feedback loops. By identifying, isolating, and supporting individuals who have been exposed to a contagious disease, public health officials can prevent further transmission, reducing the spread of the disease.

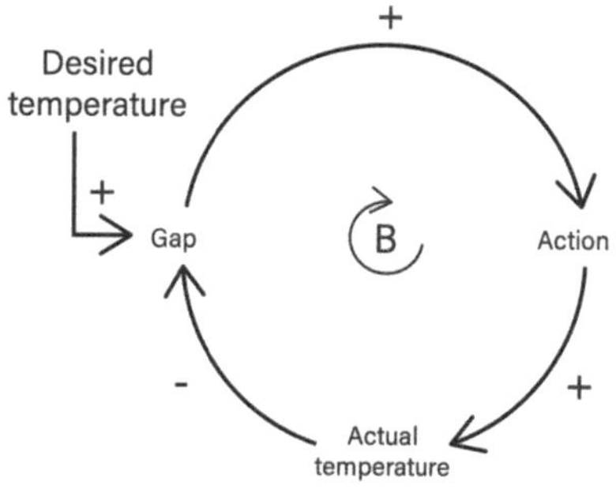

Note: A "+" or a "−" in the loop diagram indicates the nature of the action (increase or decrease). A "R" with an arrow around it is the symbol used to denote a reinforcing loop. A "B" with an arrow around it is the symbol used to denote a balancing loop.

Figure 1-2. Balancing Loop

When describing feedback loops, it is important to remember that the term *positive* refers to the amplification or increase of an outcome, and *negative* refers to diminished or decreased effect. These terms do not describe the intrinsic or moral value of an outcome but rather the increase or decrease that is the result of the looped relationship. A "+" or a "−" in the loop diagram indicates the nature of the action (increase or decrease). A "R" with an arrow around it is the symbol used to denote a reinforcing loop. A "B" with an arrow around it is the symbol used to denote a balancing loop (see Figures 1-1 and 1-2).

Balancing Feedback Loops

A balancing feedback loop is used to describe a stabilizing process within a system. A classic example of a balancing feedback loop is the way a thermostat works in a heating or cooling system to maintain a stable room temperature (Figure 1-2). When the temperature in a room deviates from the set point (desired temperature), the thermostat detects this change. If the room gets too cold, the heating system is activated to warm the room. If the room gets too hot, the cooling system is activated to cool the room. The thermostat continuously monitors the temperature and adjusts the heating or cooling to maintain the desired temperature. As a result, the temperature remains relatively stable around the set point.

Balancing feedback loops are crucial for maintaining stability in various systems.[1–3] They help prevent extreme deviations and promote resilience by continuously adjusting the system's state in response to changes or disturbances. In systems thinking, understanding the role of balancing feedback loops is essential for analyzing and designing systems with desired behaviors and outcomes. Examples of balancing feedback loops in public health include the following:

1. Immunization programs: As more individuals in a population become immunized against a contagious disease, the likelihood of an outbreak decreases. Increased

immunization rates lead to a decrease in the number of susceptible individuals, reducing the spread of the disease, which in turn encourages more people to get vaccinated.

2. Antibiotic resistance: The overuse of antibiotics can lead to antibiotic resistance, making infections harder to treat with available medication. When antibiotic resistance increases, healthcare providers become more cautious about prescribing antibiotics, and this caution slows the development of resistance.
3. Food safety regulations: Stringent regulations and inspections in food service establishments can prevent foodborne illnesses. Improved food safety practices lead to a decrease in the number of foodborne illnesses. As a result, there may be a perception that regulations can be relaxed, which can lead to lax enforcement of regulations and an increase in food safety incidents.

Feedback loops have important implications for understanding the behavior of systems. Reinforcing feedback loops create cycles of growth (virtuous) or decline (vicious), while balancing feedback loops create cycles of stability or equilibrium. Understanding the feedback loops at play within a system can help identify leverage points for intervention and design more effective policies or strategies.[6]

Causal Loop Diagrams

A causal loop diagram (CLD) is a systems thinking tool that is used to illustrate relationships between various components within a system. A CLD includes variables, arrows, polarity indicators, and the two main types of feedback loops described previously (reinforcing and balancing). Variables represent key elements in the system. Arrows represent the causal relationship between variables with arrows pointing from the influencing variable to the influenced variable. Polarities are represented by a "+" or "–". The following are some public health examples of CLDs:

Obesity Prevention

- Variables: Healthy eating, physical activity, obesity rates, education programs.
- Loops: A reinforcing loop may depict how healthy eating and regular physical activity contribute to lower obesity rates, and lower obesity rates may, in turn, lead to more encouragement for healthy behaviors. Additionally, a balancing loop may represent how increased obesity rates may prompt the development of more health education programs, which could then contribute to a reduction in obesity rates.

Infectious Disease Control

- Variables: Vaccination rates, disease prevalence, public awareness, healthcare infrastructure.

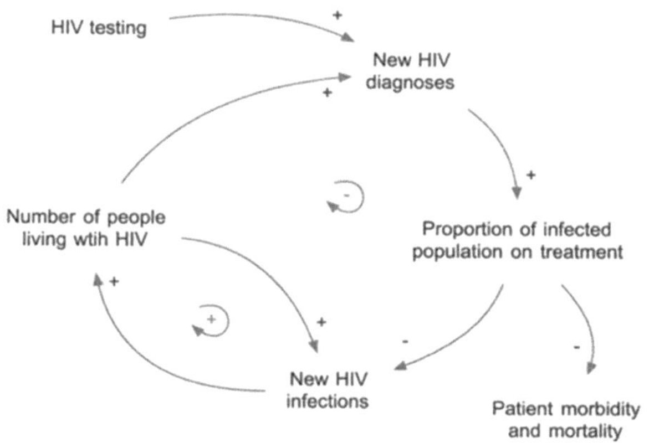

Source: Kok et al.[7] Reprinted under the terms of the CC BY license (https://creativecommons.org/licenses/by/4.0).

Figure 1-3. Causal Loop Diagram of HIV Care Continuum

- Loops: A reinforcing loop could show how high vaccination rates lead to lower disease prevalence which, in turn, encourages more people to get vaccinated. A balancing loop might depict how an increase in disease prevalence prompts public health campaigns and improved healthcare infrastructure, ultimately contributing to a decrease in disease prevalence.

Tobacco Control

- Variables: Smoking rates, tobacco cessation campaigns, tax policies and revenue, health outcomes.
- Loops: A reinforcing loop might illustrate how successful anti-smoking campaigns lead to decreased smoking rates, resulting in better health outcomes and reinforcing the effectiveness of the campaigns. Conversely, a balancing loop could represent how declining smoking rates might reduce public funding through reduced tobacco taxes for anti-smoking campaigns, potentially leading to an increase in smoking rates.

Access to Maternal and Child Health Services

- Variables: Prenatal care, maternal health, child development, and parenting education programs.
- Loops: A reinforcing loop could demonstrate how adequate prenatal care contributes to better maternal health, which, in turn, positively affects child development. Similarly, a balancing loop might illustrate how increased parenting education programs may lead to better education for parents, potentially improving care and creating a virtuous cycle.

Figure 1-3 presents an example of using feedback loops to illustrate the continuum of HIV care from testing to treatment.[7] In this figure, several individual feedback loops are

Box 1-1. Lee County Local Health District Case Study Example

The Resilience Catalysts in Public Health initiative led by researchers at George Washington University's Center for Community Resilience (CCR) is using systems thinking to eliminate community adversity and foster equity through policy, program, and practice change. As one of the first national initiatives in public health to use systems thinking to address chronic and complex social problems, the CCR team is integrating causal loop diagrams into a strategy development and action planning process to build community resilience.

The local health department (LHD) in Lee County, Iowa, is a member of the third cohort of Resilience Catalysts in Public Health sites. Lee County is a nonmetropolitan county in Southeast Iowa, bordering the Mississippi River. The estimated county population is just under 33,000 people, and the manufacturing industry dominates the employment landscape.[8] After conducting a root cause analysis to explore the historical and current factors driving inequities, Lee County's LHD team chose to focus their Resilience Catalyst initiative on improving working conditions (including access to living wages and benefits, family-friendly workplace policies, and workplace safety) and child well-being (understood as increased family economic stability and reduced child abuse and neglect).

In March 2023, the LHD hosted a group model building session (GMB), facilitated by the Center for Community Resilience. Participating community members represented mental and behavioral health services, regional planning, education, youth and family services, and equity-focused community-based organizations. During the GMB session, participants built shared understanding by defining the focus issues and mapping the system of causes and effects influencing working conditions and child well-being in Lee County. Based on causal pathways discussed during the GMB session, CCR researchers synthesized the causal loop diagram seen in Figure 1-4.

Lee County's LHD aims to use the CLD as a communications tool to shift the narrative around working conditions and child well-being. During root cause analysis, the LHD identified a reductive narrative suggesting that low labor force participation in Lee County results from community members' lack of interest in available jobs, or unwillingness to remain in the formal job market altogether. Findings from the GMB challenge this narrative. Thus, the LHD team seeks to partner with economic development and employers to increase labor force participation by creating conditions that help parents stay in the job market and take care of their families.

CCR researchers identified four main themes explaining drivers of labor force participation and visualized these in the CLD. These themes describe the interconnectedness of working conditions and family-friendly workplace policies, access to mental and behavioral health services, recruitment and retention of childcare providers, and child safety and well-being. The LHD team practiced utilizing the CLD to build a more holistic narrative around workplace policies, childcare, and health outcomes, for example:

- Parents need adequate childcare support to fully engage in the workforce. However, access to formal childcare is constrained by the lack of available childcare providers in Lee County.
- Childcare provider recruitment and retention is in turn limited by the salaries and benefits offered to childcare employees.
- Inflexible absence policies and mandatory overtime practice in the workplace (established in response to a perceived lack of workers) push parents out of the labor force, especially when they are not able to secure childcare.
- When absence policies are inflexible, parents without a robust support network or access to formal care may feel forced to settle for suboptimal or inadequate care, increasing the risk of child abuse or neglect.
- Poor working conditions lead to exhaustion and hopelessness, which in turn threaten mental health and safety, and subsequently impact employee retention.

(Continued)

Box 1-1 ***(Continued)***

- Workers, including parents, may cope with poor mental health through self-medicating, thereby increasing the risk of substance use and dependency. Low access to insurance coverage, and limited availability of in network mental and behavioral health providers heighten the risk of downstream impacts, including reduced labor force participation.
- Concurrently, exposure to substances and poor parental mental health further endanger child safety and well-being.

In addition to leveraging the summary CLD as a narrative change tool, the LHD team used insights from the CLD to determine desired outcomes for their Resilience Catalysts initiative. Examples of these outcomes include the following: employers adopting more flexible absence policies, increasing employer support for childcare, establishing recovery friendly workplaces, and increasing wage levels. The LHD team added these outcomes to their Resilience Catalysts logic model to inform action planning.

Source: A. Luisi, MA, D-K. Chen, DrPH, MPH, and W. Ellis, DrPH, MPH; Center for Community Resilience, George Washington University; unpublished report; December 24, 2023. Reprinted with permission.
Note: CCR = Center for Community Resilience; CLD = causal loop diagram; GMB = group model building; LHD = local health district.

nested together to illustrate some of the relationships between components of an HIV care system. HIV testing has a positive effect on identifying new HIV diagnoses in a community that might have been undiagnosed without the test. Identifying new HIV diagnoses leads to more HIV-positive individuals in the population being treated. The proportion of individuals with HIV on treatment reduces new HIV infections and HIV morbidity and mortality. The new HIV infections component leads to an increase in the number of individuals living with HIV, which contributes to increases in new HIV diagnoses and new HIV infections.

Of course, this is a brief depiction of a larger and more complicated HIV care system.[7] What is not included here are all the relationships between the components, including the factors that may be leading to increases in new HIV infections, such as funding for public health outreach or adherence to pre-exposure prophylaxis medications. However, the figure does demonstrate the relationships between system parts such as testing, treatment, and HIV infection, and allows for examination of their interplay within this system.

Case Study: Center for Community Resilience Causal Loop Diagram

A case study of how CLDs can be used in public health comes from the work of researchers at the Center for Community Resilience at the Milken Institute School of Public Health. The Lee County CLD case study shared in Box 1-1 illustrates how CLDs

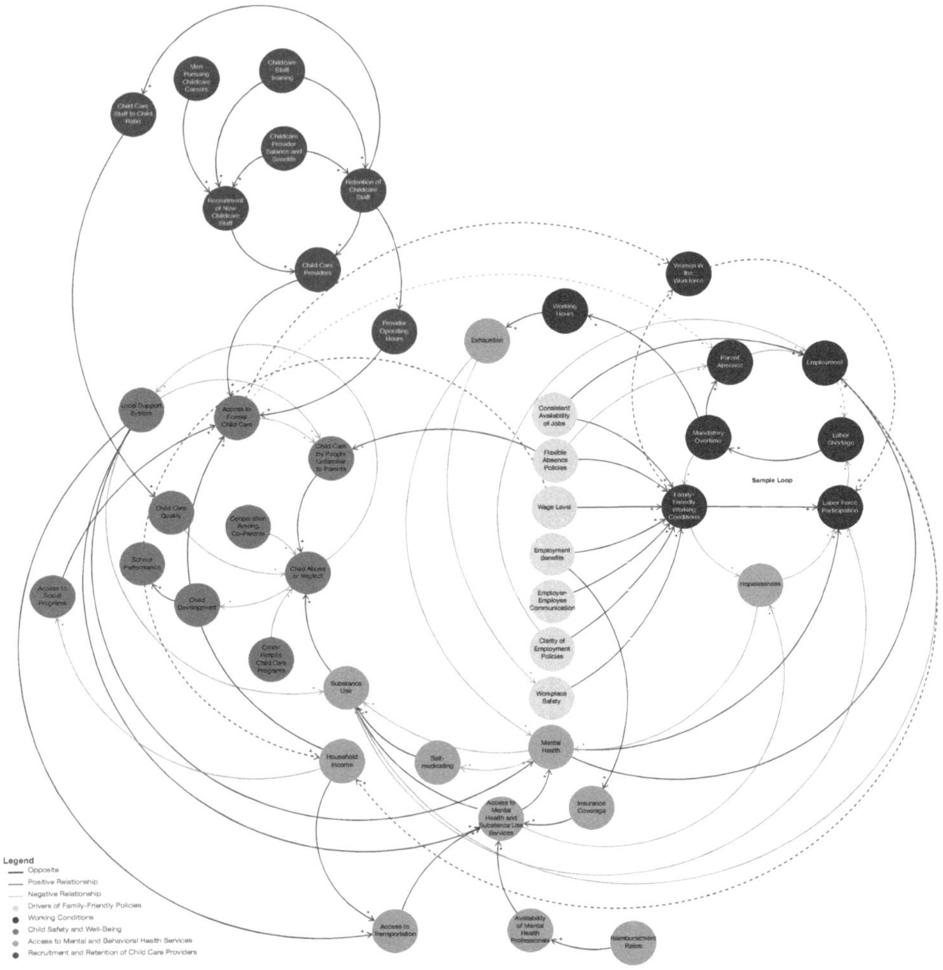

Note: See full size image at https://ajph.aphapublications.org/systems/F1-4.
Source: A. Luisi, MA, D-K. Chen, DrPH, MPH, and W. Ellis, DrPH, MPH; Center for Community Resilience, George Washington University; unpublished report; December 24, 2023. Reprinted with permission.

Figure 1-4. Causal Loop Diagram, Lee County Local Health District

can be used to address complex public health problems.[8] In this case study, a CLD was used to analyze the employment system in Lee County. The diagram helped the community see that the shortage of labor force participation was not primarily a result of individual lack of interest in securing employment but rather a complex set of related factors that made it extremely difficult to participate in the labor force, especially for low wage jobs. The CLD helped spur conversations about community resources and

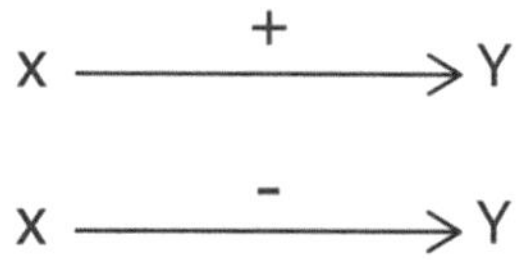

Figure 1-5. Simple Cause-and-Effect Relationship

employer efforts to support labor force participation and revealed barriers to employment that involved multiple public agencies and private entities.

Cause-and-Effect Relationships

Systems thinkers in public health can examine cause-and-effect relationships within the context of a system's other feedback loops and relationships. Figure 1-5 illustrates a simple cause-and-effect relationship, and Figure 1-6 depicts a more complex cause-and-effect relationship. Cause-and-effect relationships can be nested within larger systems diagrams that may include various feedback loops. Some examples of cause-and-effect relationships in public health include the following:

The Obesity Epidemic

- Cause: Increased consumption of high-calorie, low-nutrient foods, and decreased physical activity.
- Effect: Rising rates of obesity and related health issues, such as diabetes and cardiovascular diseases.

Infectious Disease Outbreaks

- Cause: A high number of unvaccinated individuals in a community.
- Effect: Outbreaks of vaccine-preventable diseases, such as measles or mumps.

Tobacco Use

- Cause: The availability and marketing of tobacco products.
- Effect: Increased rates of smoking-related illnesses, such as cancer or heart disease.

Climate Change and Its Impact on Health

- Cause: Greenhouse gas emissions and environmental degradation.
- Effect: Health impacts like heat-related illnesses, changes in disease patterns, and increased foodborne and waterborne diseases.

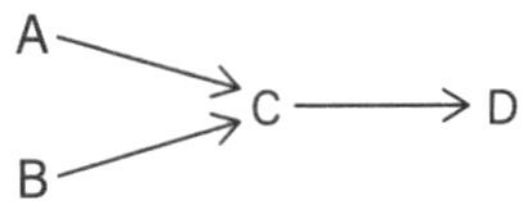

Figure 1-6. Complex Cause-and-Effect Relationship

Lead Exposure

- Cause: Exposure to lead-based paint and/or contaminated drinking water.
- Effect: Negative neurological and developmental effects in children, including learning disabilities and behavioral issues.

It is important to recognize that these cause-and-effect relationships are not isolated events, but are parts of a larger system comprised of many other relationships. Changes in one part of the system have ripple effects throughout the system and impact other components. Systems thinking helps public health professionals understand these interdependencies and design more effective interventions and policies to address them. For example, in the Lee County LHD Case Study (Box 1-1), the narrative that lack of individual interest in jobs was the cause of low labor force participation was predominant in the community. This narrative blamed individuals for not wanting to work, even though a systems approach demonstrated there were many other factors contributing to the lack of labor force participation in Lee County. The CLD demonstrated that other factors, such as available childcare and transportation, were also part of the system and tied to the cause-and-effect relationship driving the common narrative.

Stock-and-Flow Diagrams

Stock-and-flow diagrams are graphical representations that illustrate the accumulations and transfers of resources within a system, showing how inputs and outputs affect the level of stocks over time. A stock is a quantity that accumulates or depletes over time, while a flow is a rate of change that affects the level of a stock. In public health systems, examples of stocks include the following: a certain population of individuals, disease prevalence, available funding, or vaccine coverage. Example flows include the number of births or deaths, funding amounts, incidence rates, treatment rates, vaccination rates, or vaccination effectiveness rates in certain groups.

Stock-and-flow diagrams represent these relationships graphically, using boxes to represent stocks and arrows to represent flows.[1,4] The direction of the arrows indicates the direction of the flow, and the thickness of the arrow represents the magnitude of the flow.[1] A classic example of a stock-and-flow diagram is a bathtub. Figure 1-7 depicts a

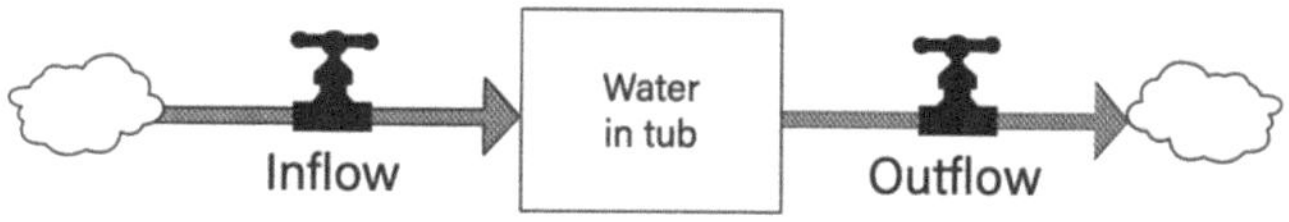

Figure 1-7. Stock-and-Flow Diagram: The Bathtub Example

stock-and-flow diagram of a bathtub that shows the water level (the stock), the faucet (the inflow), and the drain (the outflow).[1,6]

Stock-and-flow diagrams are useful tools for understanding the dynamics of systems and identifying feedback loops and other patterns of behavior. For public health systems thinkers, they can be used to explore the consequences of different policies or interventions, and to identify leverage points for intervention by adjusting quantities of a stock or adjusting rates of flow. The stock-and-flow diagram in Figure 1-8 illustrates the stock of healthy individuals flowing into at-risk populations in a community. The diagram makes clear the goal of public health interventions, which is to prevent or delay the stock of healthy and safe individuals from becoming at risk of developing a chronic disease, and if they do flow into the at-risk stock, to return them to the healthy and safe population.

Stock-and-flow diagrams can help illustrate the accumulation (stock) and movement (flow) of various elements within a system. Here are some additional examples of stock-and-flow diagrams in public health:

Infectious Disease Transmission

- Stocks: susceptible population, infected population, recovered population.
- Flows: infection rate (from susceptible to infected), recovery rate (from infected to recovered), and transmission rate (infectious contact between susceptible and infected).

Smoking Cessation Program

- Stocks: smokers, exsmokers, nonsmokers.
- Flows: smoking cessation rate (from smokers to ex-smokers), relapse rate (from ex-smokers to smokers), and population growth.

Environmental Pollution and Health Outcomes

- Stock: polluted environment, clean environment, health outcomes.
- Flows: pollution rate (from clean to polluted environment), remediation rate (from polluted to clean environment), and disease rate (from polluted environment to health outcomes).

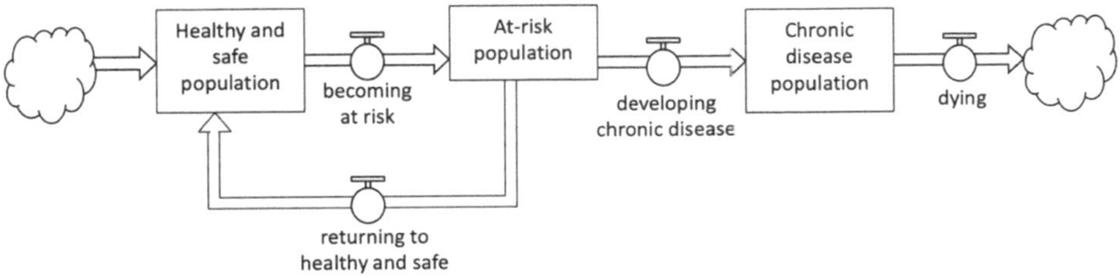

Source: J. Branscomb, MPH, Georgia Health Policy Center, PowerPoint presentation. Reprinted with permission of Georgia Health Policy Center.

Figure 1-8. Chronic Disease Stock-and-Flow Diagram

Manteuffel and colleagues developed a map of the opioid system using stock-and-flow diagrams to illustrate the relationships between parts of the system including pain treatment, prescriptions, treatment and recovery, misuse, and incarceration/justice system (Figure 1-9).[9(p161)] The map shows the complex relationships between various component parts across the opioid system.

Behavior-Over-Time Graphs

Behavior-over-time graphs are tools that systems thinkers can use to examine the behavior of systems over time. Because the outcomes of systems can be seasonal (such as disease transmission by month) and can increase and decrease over time (such as population rates or chronic disease prevalence), graphical representations that illustrate how variables within a system interact over a specific duration or period are helpful to view system behaviors and outcomes. These graphs provide a dynamic view of system evolution, allowing systems thinkers to observe trends, patterns, and the impact of various factors over time. By examining the graphical representation of variables and their interactions, systems thinkers can identify patterns, detect anomalies, and make informed decisions regarding the management and improvement of systems.

In public health, a behavior-over-time graph can be used to visualize the dynamics of a specific health indicator or variable over a given period of time (Figure 1-10). One example is the spread of a contagious disease (number of reported cases) over time. Features of this contagious disease behavior-over-time graph include the following:

- **X-axis (horizontal)**: Time
- **Y-axis (vertical)**: Number of reported cases
- **Initial state**: At the beginning of the timeline, there are few or no reported cases of the infectious disease.

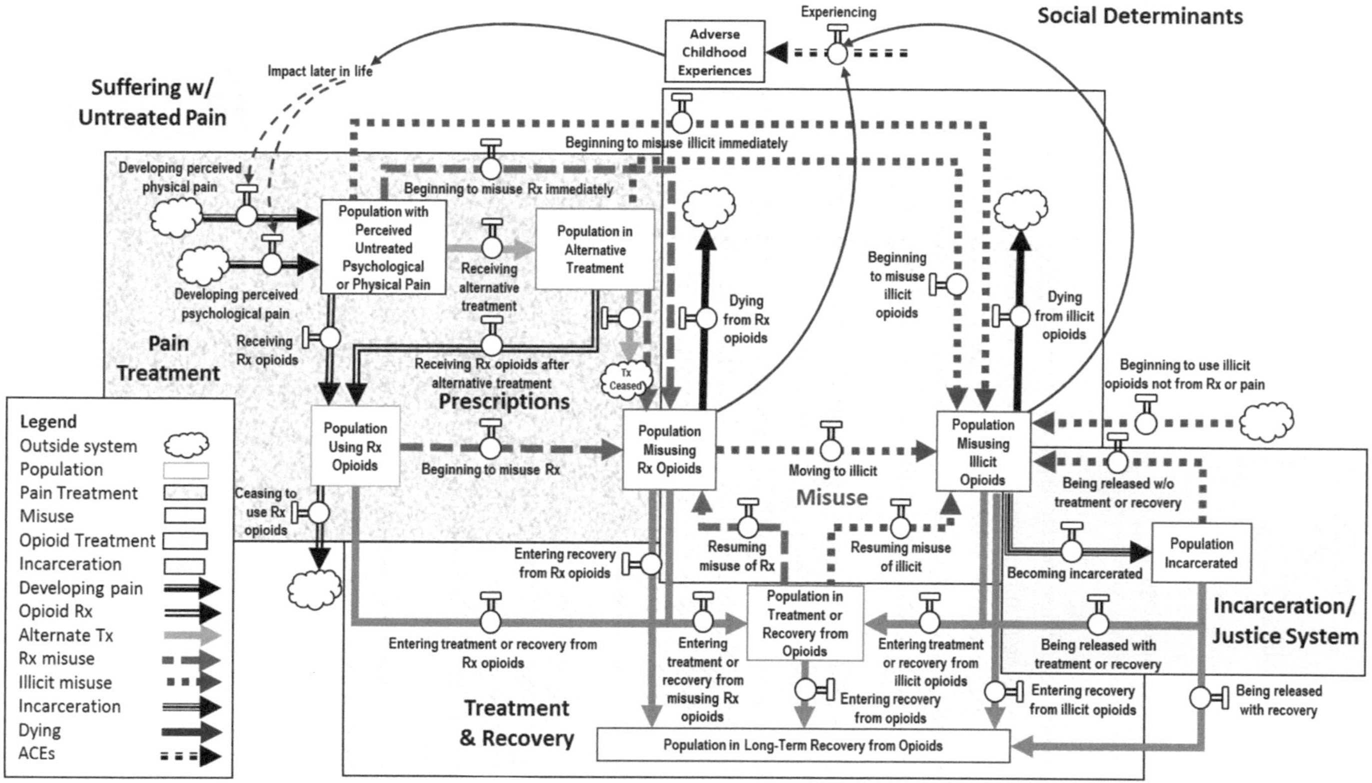

Source: Manteuffel et al.[9] Reprinted with permission of Georgia Health Policy Center and Oxford University Press (https://global.oup.com/academic/product/a-public-health-guide-to-ending-the-opioid-epidemic-9780190056810)

Note: ACE = adverse childhood experience; Rx = prescription; Tx = treatment.

Figure 1-9. Opioid System Map

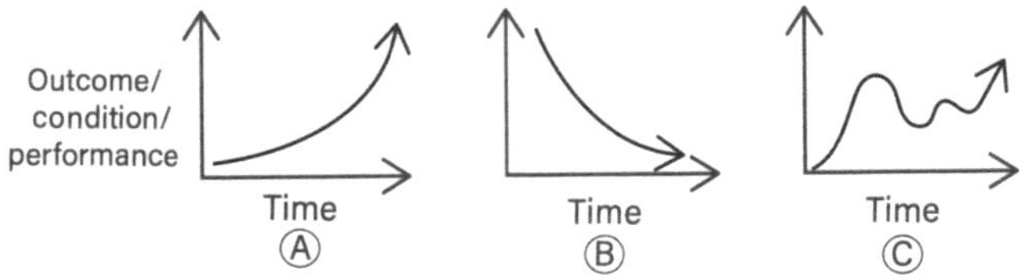

Figure 1-10. Behavior-Over-Time Diagrams

- **Outbreak period**: As the disease starts spreading, the graph would show a rising trend, indicating an increasing number of reported cases over time (Figure 1-10, graph A).
- **Public health interventions**: When public health interventions are implemented (e.g., vaccination campaigns, quarantine measures, public awareness programs), the graph shows a change in the slope, in this case a slow of the rate of decrease (Figure 1-10, graph B).
- **Peak incidence**: There might be a point where the number of reported cases reaches a peak, indicating the highest point of disease incidence during the outbreak.
- **Possible resurgence** (second wave): In some cases, there might be a resurgence or second wave of cases if control measures are lifted prematurely or if the disease has the potential to re-emerge (Figure 1-10, graph C).
- **Sustained control**: A successful public health intervention would ideally lead to a sustained decrease in the number of reported cases over an extended period.

Behavior-over-time graphs can help public health officials, policymakers, and researchers understand the impact of interventions, identify trends, and make informed decisions. They also allow for the exploration of feedback loop behaviors, such as how public awareness campaigns may influence behavior and subsequently impact disease transmission rates over time.

Advanced systems thinking techniques like simulation models can be used to assess options for mitigation and observe differences between various interventions over time. Calancie and colleagues describe the use of behavior-over-time graphs in their article where they provide a behavior-over-time graph that depicts per capita annual cigarette consumption in the US by major interventions that impacted cigarette consumption at various points in history (Figure 1-11).[10]

Mindsets and System Behavior: The Iceberg Metaphor

The iceberg metaphor is an analogy often used in systems thinking to illustrate the visible and less visible aspects of complex systems.[1,11,12] This metaphor helps systems thinkers visualize the importance of looking beyond the surface-level components of a system to delve deeper into behaviors, attitudes, and structures that are parts of a system.[11,12]

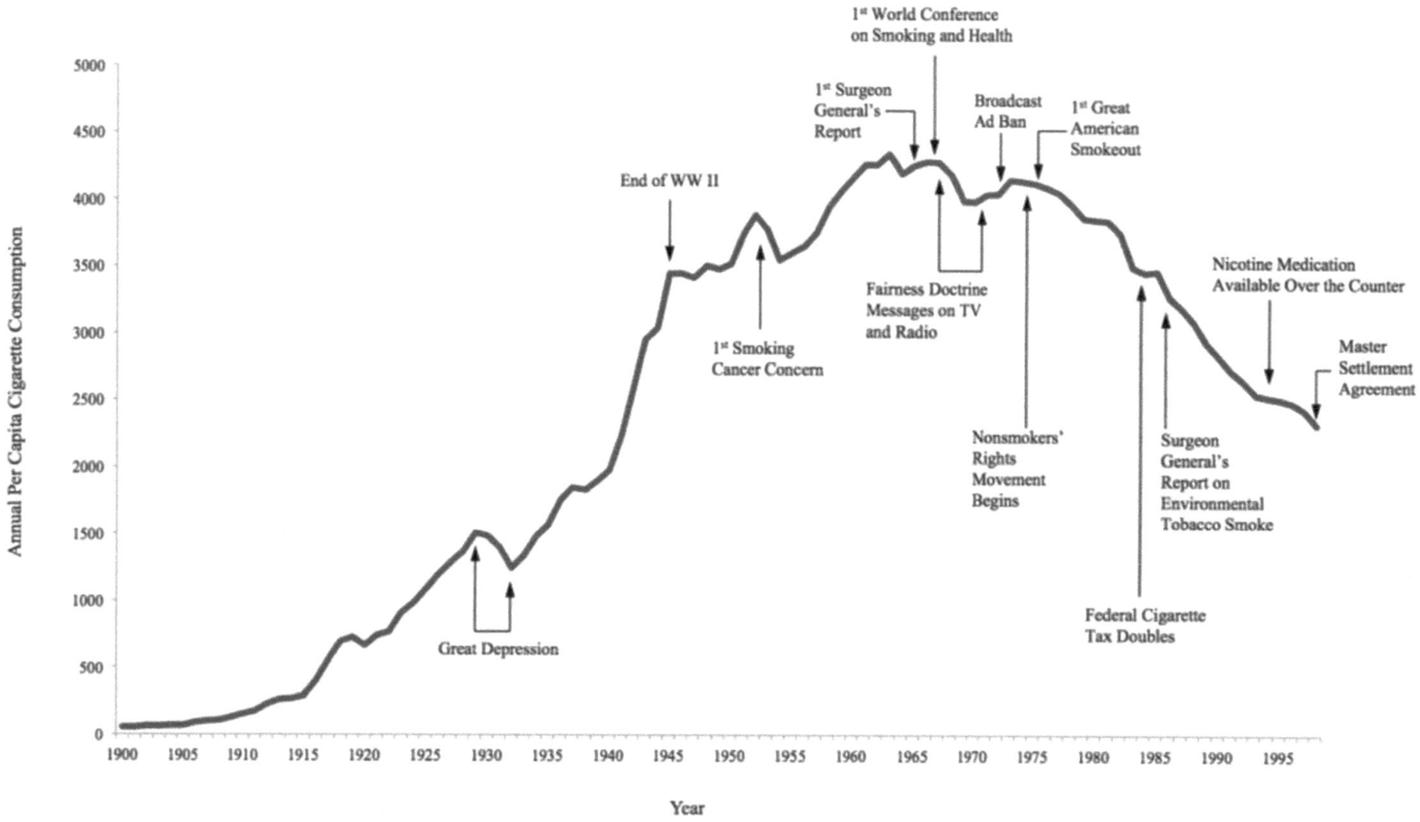

Source: Reprinted from Calancie et al.[10]

Figure 1-11. Annotated Behavior-Over-Time Graph, Cigarette Consumption by Year

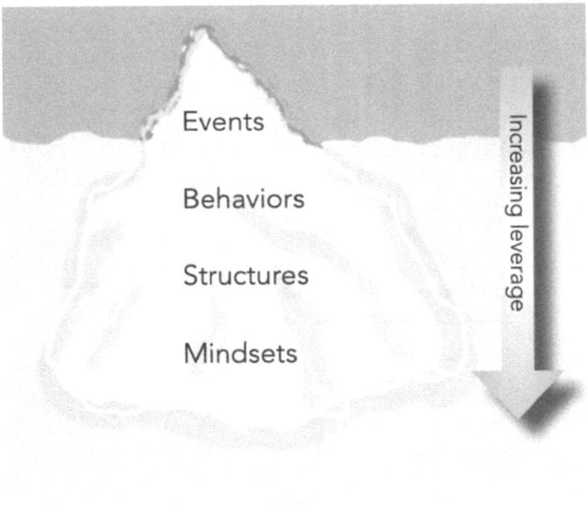

The Iceberg, a metaphor for the level at which individuals interact with a system.

Source: Reprinted with permission of Georgia Health Policy Center.[12]

Figure 1-12. The Iceberg Metaphor in Systems Thinking

The iceberg metaphor is based on the idea that an iceberg floating in the ocean consists of a visible portion above the waterline and a much larger, hidden, portion below the ocean's surface (Figure 1-12). The part of the iceberg above the water line represents the observable aspects of a problem. These are the clearly visible and explicit parts of a system, such as events and observable system behaviors. The submerged part of the iceberg symbolizes underlying, less visible parts of a system such as mindsets, attitudes, and structures that have a large impact on system behavior but are not clearly visible when looking at the system's most obvious components.

Addressing only the visible symptoms (the tip of the iceberg) may fail to resolve the root causes of the problem that are often hidden below the surface but have significant impact on the system's results. When looking at a system using the iceberg metaphor, systems thinkers can ask the following questions:

- Looking at the visible or "tip of the iceberg" events:
    - What has happened in the system?
    - What do we observe?
- Looking at the "below the water" factors:
    - What behaviors are part of the system?
    - What is happening in terms of system trends and behaviors over time?
    - What structures influence behaviors, including policies and laws?
    - What mental models, including assumptions or beliefs, are part of the system?

The iceberg metaphor encourages systems thinkers to go beyond analyzing the easily visible parts of a system to explore the underlying structures, mindsets, and behaviors that drive complex systems. By doing so, they can gain a deeper understanding of the dynamics at play and make more informed decisions when seeking to improve or intervene in a system.

Examples of Systems Thinking in Public Health

There are many ways that systems thinking can be used in public health. The examples that follow demonstrate the breadth of systems thinking as an approach to two public health challenges: obesity prevention and tobacco control.

The Obesity System

The obesity epidemic is a complex issue that involves a range of social, economic, environmental, and individual factors. Applying systems thinking to understanding obesity can help public health professionals identify the drivers of obesity and develop more effective interventions. Systems thinking can be used to understand the complex interrelationships between social, economic, and environmental factors that influence obesity rates. It can be used to map the food environment and understand how food choices and eating behaviors are driven by many different factors and contribute to changes in other parts of the obesity system.

The obesity system CLD shown in Figure 1-13 was developed by Allender and colleagues and illustrates the complicated nature of the drivers of obesity and the numerous points of intervention that can be leveraged to support change.[13(p8)] As such, public health professionals must work across professional sectors and governmental departments to approach obesity as a complex problem requiring multiple levels of intervention. Sectors that would be included are education departments, recreation and environmental planning agencies, families and community groups, as well as the private sector actors across the food system.

In the obesity CLD, we see the main components of the obesity system, including general physical activity, participation in sport, fast food and junk food availability, and social influences. Within these components are feedback loops and relationships between parts that influence obesity rates. Cause-and-effect relationships and causal loops illustrate reinforcing and balancing relationships throughout the system. Systems thinkers would then engage in discussions and analysis of what leverage points may yield the most improvement in lowering obesity rates in the community. These leverage points become the basis for public health action.

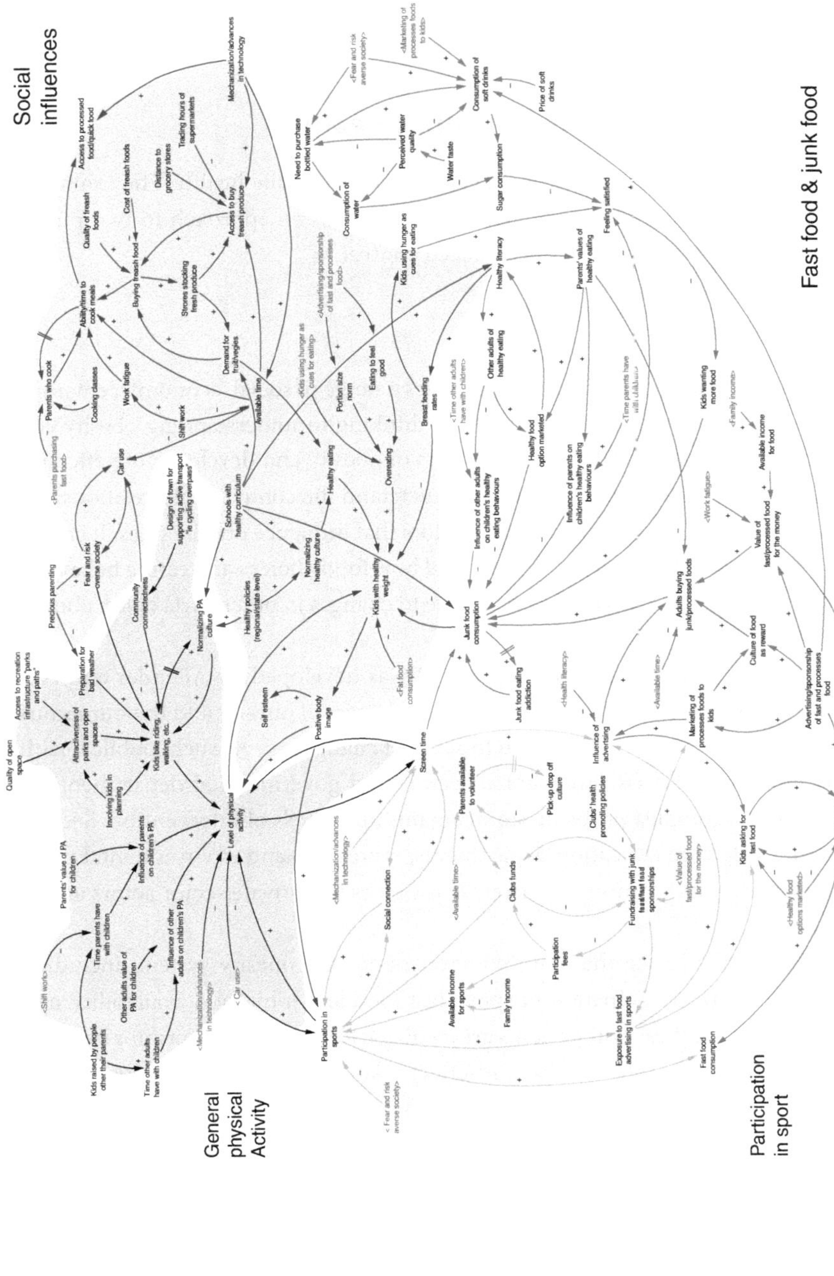

Note: See full size image at https://ajph.aphapublications.org/systems/F1-13.

Source: Allender et al.[13(p8)] Reprinted under the terms of the CC BY license (https://creativecommons.org/licenses/by/4.0).

Figure 1-13. Causal Loop Diagram of the Causes of Childhood Obesity in a Community

The Tobacco Control System

Applying systems thinking to tobacco control helps public health practitioners address the complex and multifaceted factors that contribute to tobacco use. Systems thinking can be used to examine the way that the tobacco industry influences the tobacco control system, through behaviors including marketing, lobbying, and product innovation. Systems thinking can also be used to see how social norms around smoking and changes over time in the social acceptability of tobacco use influence outcomes. CLDs can be used to understand the complex interrelationships between addiction, mental health, and smoking behavior. This approach supports interventions that address the root causes of smoking behavior across the system.

A causal map of the tobacco control system (Figure 1-14) developed by staff at the National Cancer Institute presents a graphical way to assess the tobacco control system and intervention opportunities.[14(p125)] In this system, we see the complicated relationships between the many parts of the tobacco control system, including public health efforts, industry behaviors, government structures and policies, and individual behaviors. This map demonstrates the many points of leverage at which an effective and comprehensive tobacco control campaign can intervene to successfully reduce tobacco use in a population. These leverage points include policies that limit marketing of tobacco, funding for health research, and changing social norms around smoking.[14]

CHANGING PUBLIC HEALTH SYSTEMS BY IDENTIFYING LEVERAGE POINTS

As described in the previous sections, achieving meaningful change in public health requires a deep understanding of the underlying systems, their components, and the leverage points that can be manipulated to drive public health outcomes. According to Meadows, a leverage point is a specific element within a system where a change or intervention can lead to an effect on the overall system.[15] Meadows' 12 leverage points for systems change provide valuable insight into how to address public health challenges effectively.[15] Each of these leverage points can be used to create potential change in a system.

Meadows ranked these 12 leverage points in terms of the magnitude of change that could be obtained from each.[15] These 12 points are presented in rank order from highest impact to lowest impact, as follows.

1. The power to transcend paradigms: Transcending paradigms means shifting fundamental mindsets or worldviews about what is "true".[15(p19)] Meadows suggests that this involves moving beyond existing mental models and embracing new ways of thinking beyond known paradigms when looking at systems.[15] This leverage point encourages us to challenge established beliefs and explore alternative approaches to problem-solving within a system. To achieve the most impact in a system and transcend

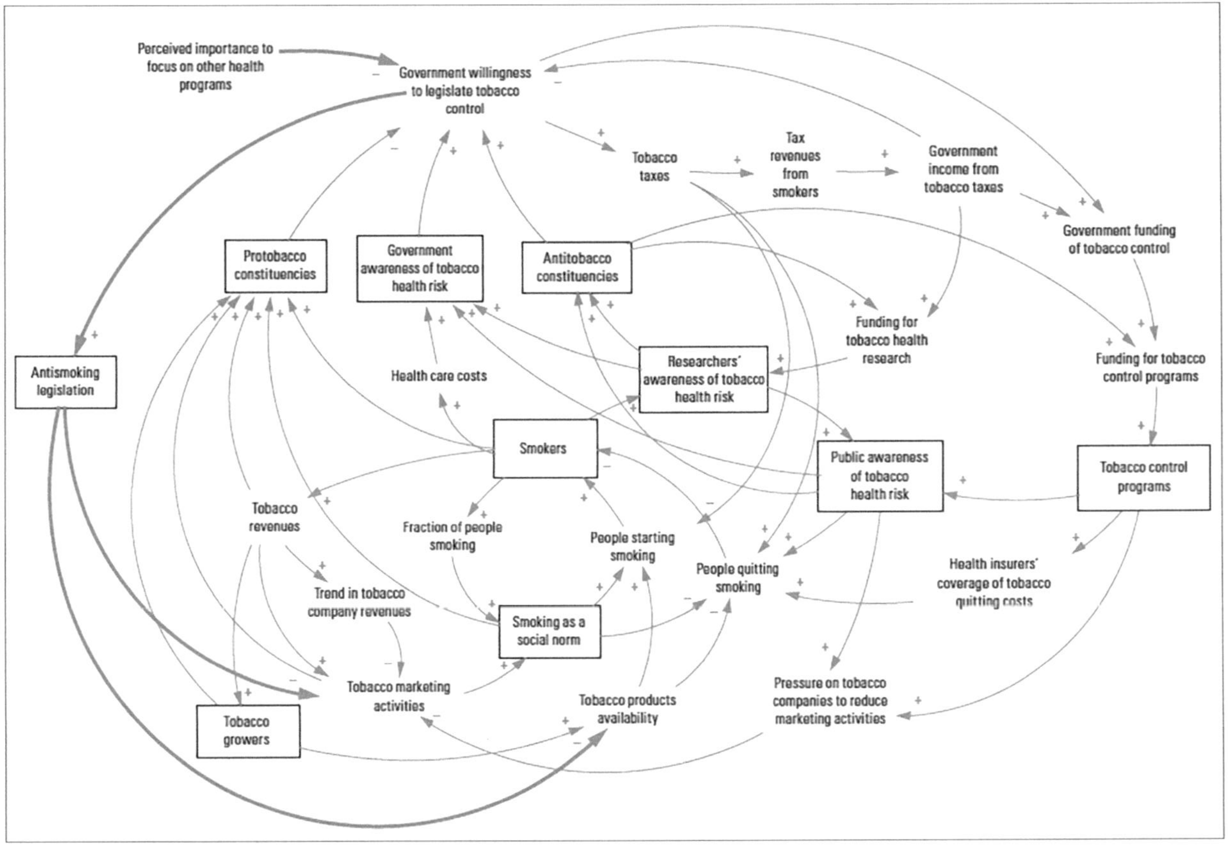

Source: Reprinted from National Cancer Institute.[14(p125)]

Figure 1-14. The Tobacco System Causal Map Example

paradigms in public health, practitioners can shift from fragmented and reactive approaches to public health problems to holistic and proactive ones. By adopting paradigms that prioritize prevention, equity, and community engagement and empowerment, public health efforts can become more effective and sustainable.

2. The mindset or paradigm out of which the system arises: The mindset or paradigm leverage point refers to the overarching belief system, values, and assumptions that shape a system.[15] It forms the foundation upon which the system's goals, rules, structure, and parameters are built. Changing mindsets can lead to profound shifts in the entire system's behavior and outcomes. Public health systems are shaped by the prevailing paradigms. Shifting the paradigm to one that emphasizes prevention, health promotion, and social determinants of health can lead to more comprehensive and equitable health outcomes. The way that the Lee County LHD analysis shifted the dominant narrative around labor force participation is a good example of this leverage point.
3. The goals of the system: The goals of a system determine its purpose and direction.[15] By redefining and realigning system goals, we can influence a system's behavior to prioritize different outcomes. For instance, shifting from profit-driven goals to goals oriented toward improving well-being can transform an entire system's dynamics. Aligning the goals of the public health system with the well-being of individuals and communities is crucial. Prioritizing objectives such as reducing health disparities, improving access to healthcare, and enhancing overall well-being are goal-changing leverage points that can drive better outcomes.
4. The power to add, change, evolve, or self-organize system structure: This leverage point focuses on the ability to modify the structural components and relationships within a system.[15] By adding, changing, or allowing elements of the structure to self-organize, we can adapt the system to better meet its intended objectives or to respond to changing conditions. The ability to add or change structures within the system can enable rapid responses to emerging health threats and evolving community needs. Innovations in healthcare delivery, technology, and policy can enhance a system's resilience and effectiveness. Changing technology, for example artificial intelligence (AI), could dramatically change the public health workforce's daily activities and how leaders staff governmental public health agencies. Using policy to change structural relationships, such expanding who has access to public health services, can also lead to structural changes in a system and better health outcomes.
5. The rules of the system: Rules, including incentives, punishments, and constraints, define how individuals and entities within a system behave.[15] Modifying a system's rules can alter the incentives and disincentives that drive behavior, influencing the overall system's performance. The rules governing public health programs, including public health regulations and policies, play a significant role in shaping health outcomes. Designing and implementing rules that encourage healthy behaviors can lead to positive system change.

6. The structure of information flows: Information flows are the channels through which data, knowledge, and communication move within a system.[15] Using this leverage point to restructure how information flows can impact decision-making processes, accessibility to information, and the distribution of power within a system. Effective public health relies on accurate and timely population data. Ensuring equitable access to information, and promoting transparency and equity in data collection, analysis, and dissemination, empowers communities and stakeholders to make informed decisions and participate in shaping health policies. Changing who sees what data, for example sharing data with community members at the neighborhood versus the aggregated city level, can help communities better understand their local health assets and their challenges.
7. The gain around driving positive feedback loops: As described previously, positive feedback loops amplify and reinforce outcomes in a system.[15] Manipulating the positive gains these loops create can accelerate desired changes or dampen unwanted ones. Public health systems can benefit from reinforcing positive feedback loops. For example, by investing in early childhood education, a system can reinforce the health effects that result from more children learning earlier and more parents being able to participate in the labor force. Improving access to healthy food in a neighborhood can support efforts to increase nutrition and prevent or better manage chronic diseases. In short, system changes that reinforce better outcomes create virtuous cycles of improved health and well-being.
8. The strength of balancing feedback loops: Balancing feedback loops are stabilizing mechanisms that counteract deviations from desired states.[15] Adjusting the strength of these loops can help maintain system stability or make corrections that are more responsive to changes and disruptions. Balancing feedback loops in public health are essential for maintaining stability and addressing issues like disease outbreaks. Strengthening the capacity to detect, respond to, and control health threats is critical for minimizing harm and maintaining system resilience.
9. The lengths of delays, relative to the rate of system change: Delays in a system's response time are a leverage point that can lead to either desired or undesired consequences based on the system's outcomes.[15] Slowing disease spread would be a desired delay in a disease mitigation system. Speeding up a public health response system can improve the speed of disease diagnosis and treatment, and rapid communication can prevent the spread of misinformation or panic during a public health emergency.
10. The structure of stocks and flows: Stocks and flows pertain to the physical resources in a specific stock-and-flow relationship and their overall movement within a system.[15] Influencing stocks by increasing or decreasing flows impacts resource allocation, distribution, and utilization, and influences system behavior. The flow of resources, such as providing increased financial supports in a food program or

increasing transportation services to bring clients to public health service sites, can enhance the effectiveness of public health interventions.

11. The sizes of buffers and other stabilizing stocks: Buffers and stabilizing stocks act as reserves that absorb fluctuations in a system and maintain system stability.[15] Adjusting the sizes of these buffers can affect the system's resilience and ability to withstand shocks. Building resilient public health systems requires adequate resources and infrastructure. Maintaining a buffer of medical supplies or surge staffing for emergency response, for example, can help mitigate the impact of public health crises.
12. Constants, parameters, and numbers: These leverage points represent fixed factors that govern a system's behavior.[15] Changing these values through subsidies, taxes, or standards can have a direct and predictable impact on system dynamics. For instance, implementing sugar-sweetened beverage taxes to reduce sugar consumption, subsidizing healthy foods in a nutrition program so they are more affordable to participants, or setting air quality standards to reduce pollution-related illnesses are effective ways to leverage parameters that can lead to improved public health.

These 12 leverage points allow us to address public health challenges comprehensively and effectively. By transcending paradigms, aligning goals, and strategically manipulating other leverage points in a system, systems thinkers can work towards a healthier and more equitable future by creating lasting systems change. Meadows states that it is important to note that leverage points which change how we think (mindsets, paradigms) and how we set system goals have the most potential for systems change, and quantitative changes (constants, parameters, numbers, or the size of buffers) have the least.[15]

THE CHALLENGES OF SYSTEMS THINKING

While systems thinking has been widely adopted in various fields, it is not without its challenges and critiques. The emphasis on complexity and interconnectedness can overwhelm rather than clarify understandings of a system because systems intersect and it is often difficult to define clear boundaries between them. Systems thinking often involves the use of abstract models and diagrams which can sometimes obscure the real-world complexity of the issues being addressed in favor of a simple graphic or diagram.

There are several ways to address these challenges. First, it is important to remember that there is no one way to do systems thinking. Rather, systems thinking is an approach or perspective that uses a set of tools to help uncover complexity and connectedness, including the behaviors and mindsets that generate specific results over time. Second, it is important to involve a range of stakeholders in the process to ensure that systems thinking is comprehensive and representative of diverse perspectives. This includes engaging individuals from different sectors, disciplines, and communities who can provide unique insights into the dynamics of the system being studied. Finally, it is important to emphasize transparency and accountability in systems thinking approaches. This includes clearly articulating the assumptions and limitations of systems models and tools and providing evidence to support their validity and effectiveness.

Systems thinking requires an adaptive approach that considers the entirety of the context in which public health work is practiced. Despite the best intentions of myriad public health practitioners, if public health efforts are not clearly focused on understanding the systems in which they are working, their impact will be modest at best. The adage, "a bad system will beat a good person every time," comes to mind.[16] This is why systems thinking, and systems change, is vital to public health improvement.

REFERENCES

1. Meadows DH. *Thinking in Systems: A Primer*. Chelsea Green Publishing; 2008.
2. Rowitz L. *Public Health Leadership: Putting Principles into Action*. Jones and Bartlett Learning; 2014.
3. Branscomb J, Dills JE, Landers G, Minyard KJ, Hassmiller L. Systems thinking for public health professionals. In: Fraser MR, Castrucci CC, eds. *Building Strategic Skills for Better Health: A Primer for Public Health Professionals*. Oxford University Press; 2024:38–53.
4. Senge PM. *The Fifth Discipline: The Art and Practice of the Learning Organization*. Random House; 1990.
5. World Health Organization. National health planning tools, health system building blocks. Updated 2010. Accessed January 2, 2024. https://extranet.who.int/nhptool/BuildingBlock.aspx
6. Sterman JD. *Business Dynamics: Systems Thinking and Modeling for a Complex World*. McGraw-Hill Education; 2000.
7. Kok S, Rutherford AR, Gustafson R, Barrios R, Montaner JS, Vasarhelyi K. Optimizing an HIV testing program using a system dynamics model of the continuum of care. *Health Care Manag Sci*. 2015;18(3):334–362. doi:10.1007/s10729-014-9312-0
8. US Census Bureau. Lee County, Iowa. 2020. Accessed January 2, 2024. https://data.census.gov/profile/Lee_County,_Iowa?g=050XX00US19111
9. Manteuffel B, Alderman L, Branscomb J, Minyard K. Systems thinking and the opioid epidemic in Georgia. In: Fraser MR, Butler JC, eds. *A Public Health Guide to Ending the Opioid Epidemic*. Oxford University Press; 2019:159–170.
10. Calancie L, Anderson S, Branscomb J, Apostolico AA, Lich KH. Using behavior over time graphs to spur systems thinking among public health practitioners. *Prev Chronic Dis* 2018;15:170254. doi:10.5888/pcd15.170254
11. Bender K. Systems thinking in public health. In: Helm-Murtagh SC, Erwin P, eds. *Leadership in Practice: Essentials for Public Health and Healthcare Leaders*. Springer Publishing; 2023:33–53.
12. Georgia Health Policy Center, Georgia State University. Systems Thinking at the Georgia Health Policy Center. July 12, 2017. Accessed January 2, 2024. https://ghpc.gsu.edu/tools-frameworks/systems-thinking
13. Allender S, Owen B, Kuhlberg J, et al. A community based systems diagram of obesity causes. *PloS ONE*. 2015;10(7):e0129683. doi:10.1371/ journal.pone.0129683

14. *Greater Than the Sum: Systems Thinking in Tobacco Control.* National Cancer Institute; 2007. Tobacco Control Monograph No. 18. https://cancercontrol.cancer.gov/sites/default/files/2020-08/m18_complete.pdf
15. Meadows D. Leverage points: Places to intervene in a system. The Academy for Systems Change. 1999. Accessed January 2, 2024. https://donellameadows.org/archives/leverage-points-places-to-intervene-in-a-system
16. Hunter J. A bad system will beat a good person every time. The W. Edwards Deming Institute. Accessed January 2, 2024. https://deming.org/a-bad-system-will-beat-a-good-person-every-time

2

What Is Strategic Thinking?

Strategic thinking is the activity of analyzing complex situations, considering multiple perspectives, and generating innovative insights to address organizational challenges and opportunities. Strategic thinking focuses on developing a robust understanding of an organization's external and internal environments, and identifying trends, patterns, and potential disruptions that could impact outcomes and organizational effectiveness. Strategists use systems thinking tools to assess and understand big picture problems, and to optimally position organizational activities in the larger systems in which they operate.

As mentioned at the outset of this primer, the systems and strategic thinking skill has been identified as a professional growth area by many working in governmental public health agencies. Many in the public health workforce join their organizations as technical or subject matter experts. For example, they bring technical knowledge to their work as epidemiologists, environmental health specialists, grants administrators, and public health nurses. Over time, some of these individuals are moved into leadership positions based on their performance as technical experts. As individuals move into new public health leadership positions, there is often a need for them to develop more strategic thinking competencies because their day-to-day activities at work become less about the technical aspects of the job and more about working with people, setting organizational direction, and holding individuals accountable for results. Research conducted by strategist and author Rich Horwath suggests that executive competency in strategic thinking and strategic "acuity" are vital to successful organizational performance and longevity, more so than functional or technical knowledge.[1(p18)] While his research focused on private sector corporations, his findings are certainly applicable to nonprofit and governmental organizations where executive leaders oversee large teams and significant budgets that require strategic thinking to function well.

Given the importance of strategy to organizational success, why do we not spend more time thinking strategically in our work? In his study of 500 managers in 25 different companies, Horwath found ten key reasons or "strategy challenges" to thinking strategically.[1(p5)] Not surprisingly, time was the most common reason. In his study, 96% of all managers were so overwhelmed with doing the work that they could not make the time to think strategically about it. I have heard this reason for not thinking strategically come up in many different organizations. The question then becomes, if we are not making time to think strategically, how are we sure that our actions are strategic? Are we just busy doing things? Do we run the risk of misaligning activities and wasting effort as a result of not taking time to step back and look at the entirety of the work and the alignment of multiple efforts across the organization? Making time for strategic thinking should be a priority for every member of an organization's staff in order to ensure that individual activities support shared agency goals and that the various parts of the organization work together to reach collective priorities.

The second most frequent reason that managers in Horwath's study gave for not thinking strategically was what he terms "commitment" to the organization's strategy.[1(p6)] Staff commitment and buy-in to the organization's strategy are important; you want your team to help develop and own your organizational strategy and to understand their roles in implementing it. But the farther away staff are from the strategic planning and implementation process, the less likely they may be to buy into it, understand how it relates to their work, or to even know that a plan exists at all. This is why engaging groups of agency staff and stakeholders in the strategic thinking and planning process is important. Shared development of an agency's plan and shared tracking of progress supports staff commitment to the agency's strategic goals. Routine communication about organizational strategy from leaders and managers throughout the daily life of an organization is also essential. All staff must regularly receive updates on the agency's progress in meeting strategic goals, not only to celebrate successes but also to ensure that the agency's strategic priorities align with the efforts and activities of their work units.

In Horwath's study, managers also reported lack of priorities as a barrier to thinking strategically.[1] Clear priority setting is critical to organizational success. Everyone in an organization should understand the organization's mission, goals, and priorities. A strategy that is too broad prioritizes everything, and as a result the organization may accomplish very little. A strategy that is too narrow may limit organizational success and fail to connect efforts that have organizational value. Productive strategic thinking requires assessing these important trade-offs. Trade-offs involve making decisions about which activities will and will not continue within an organization. This can be difficult, especially in large organizations with numerous program areas that have existed for a long time. However, a clear understanding of what an organization will and will not do is essential to strategic thinking and to positioning the organization for a successful future.

Other challenges to thinking strategically identified by Horwath include the "status quo,"[1(p7)] that occurs when staff benefit from the current state and do not want to change, and when staff do not understand what a strategy is or how their work fits into it. Other challenges include lack of training and tools to think strategically, lack of goal alignment between members of the organization, "firefighting"[1(p9)] (reacting to daily developments vs. making time to think proactively about the long term), lack of data, and unclear information. It is highly likely that even if you are devoted to thinking strategically, many staff in your organization will need support in dealing with one or more of these barriers to thinking strategically in practice.

WHY DOES STRATEGIC THINKING MATTER?

Contemporary public health practice requires strategic thinking. The national report "Public Health 3.0: A Call to Action for Public Health to Meet the Challenges of the 21st Century" was released in 2017 by the US Department of Health and Human Services' Office of the Assistant Secretary for Health. This report calls on public health leaders to serve as chief health strategists for their jurisdictions.[2] In this role, public health leaders and their teams support efforts to identify strategic opportunities to cross organizational boundaries to improve health. The Assistant Secretary's "Call to Action" states the following:

> Public Health 3.0 refers to a new era of enhanced and broadened public health practice that goes beyond traditional public department functions and programs. Cross-sectoral collaboration is inherent to the Public Health 3.0 vision, and the Chief Health Strategist role requires high-achieving health organizations with the skills and capabilities to drive such collective action.[2(p3)]

Public Health 3.0 and the chief health strategist concept emphasize the need for public health leaders to think strategically about how to obtain the best health outcomes for their jurisdiction's population. While some have been critical of the chief health strategist concept, arguing that individuals in other health entities such as hospitals or health systems may also serve this role, the chief health strategist concept does not mean that other public health or health care leaders cannot think strategically about a community's health. Rather, the concept emphasizes governmental public health agencies' unique and fundamental role in assessing and developing opportunities for population health improvement that include everyone in their jurisdictions.

The chief health strategist role supports the notion that successful public health practice includes taking time to consider the alignment of priorities, goals, and resources to support an agency's work. Public Health 3.0 stresses the notion that the transformation of public health required to meet 21st-century public health problems necessitates moving away from disease-specific or categorical programs in agencies and toward solutions to health improvement based in systems and strategic thinking that cross sectors. Strategic thinking matters because it helps organizational leaders and their teams move toward these crosscutting, long-term visions and goals. In their chapter on strategic thinking in the book *Leadership in Practice*, Ginter and Duncan state that "strategic thinking is the clearest signal of the existence of leadership in an organization and it is the leaders in an organization who must be the initiators, keepers, and promoters of the vision of an organization."[3(p69)]

When an organization lacks a coherent strategy or when organizational leaders fail to effectively communicate strategy, agency staff may feel disconnected from a common purpose, may not understand why their work is significant to the organization, or may unintentionally pursue activities and efforts that duplicate the work of others. Strategy setting in governmental public health agencies is difficult because there are many interests and stakeholders involved. Strategic thinking in government goes beyond typical corporate strategy development, which is generally created and directed by an organization's corporate board of directors and implemented by organizational management.

Setting governmental public health agency strategy includes many different constituents and communities, agency staff, policymakers at many levels, funders, and stakeholders. While strategic thinking in the private and nonprofit sector is an executive and management function, strategic thinking and strategy development in government also includes legislative and diplomatic competencies because many health agencies are directed by multiple governmental oversight entities and elected leaders. These entities include boards of health, local, territorial, and state legislatures, mayors, county commissioners, city councilors, appointed leaders of large health and human service agencies, and ultimately, the public. Setting priorities and developing strategy for agencies with all these interests and influences is difficult but no less essential to organizational performance than the need for strategy in private corporations and nonprofit organizations guided by boards of directors.

Despite the complexity involved in developing governmental public health strategy, strategic thinking is an indispensable skill for governmental public health professionals. In a chapter on strategy, I noted the following:

> A public health agency's strategic plan should summarize the unique and strategic position leadership wants to take in addressing a jurisdiction's priorities. Agencies without strategy tend to be directionless, characterized by programmatic silos and little cross-agency collaboration. To inspire strategic thinking, leaders need to repeatedly share their ideas and efforts to make the multiple activities of an agency fit together and complement one another. Strategy is the foundation for all staff in all positions of the agency. Communicating strategy allows staff to obtain a coherent sense of how their work and their role helps move important goals forward and improves the health of their jurisdictions.[4(p25–26)]

Strategy, and most importantly the organization's vision and mission, are the threads that connect members of a public health organization and guide their shared work of advancing and improving health regardless of their job title, program area, or area of professional specialization. Without strategy, an organization is a collection of activities, busy people, and hopes and dreams. With strategy, organizations move toward collective priorities that energize efforts across the organization and motivate and excite staff by linking their activities with realistic and attainable goals.

Strategy and Adaptive Leadership

Strategy is also essential to assuring that an organization can respond and adapt to changes in its environment. By anticipating potential changes and identifying new opportunities that may result, strategic thinkers help organizations stay ahead of known roadblocks. Consideration of future changes helps organizational leaders avoid being caught off guard by events in the environment that might go unnoticed without strategic thinking.

While not a public health example, the demise of the Men's Dress Furnishing Association, the national group representing necktie manufacturers, is an important example of the need to think strategically and anticipate future trends. The group ultimately dissolved in 2008 after failing to adapt to the growing fashion trend of men forgoing neckties and the economic trend of men cutting their spending on clothing due to the Great Recession.[5] Certainly, the tieless trend evolved over time and the association could have seen the signals, including the fact that many attending the Association's annual luncheon themselves showed up tieless.[5] Strategic thinking could have informed the Association's strategy and strategic moves away from neckties toward new fashion trends (e.g., the growing popularity of patterned or novelty socks), and could have foretold the impact of economic changes on their members' customers.

Would strategic thinking have changed men's minds about the comfort of neckties and their necessity? Probably not. However, strategic thinking could have anticipated what this tieless trend would mean for the organization's work and helped discern the organization's position and priorities as a result. This is an allegorical example for public health leaders. How many of your organizational activities depend on old or outdated trends, and how adept is your organization at anticipating new ones? Strategic thinking can help support your efforts to assess and evaluate the impact of trends and to adapt your efforts to meet the future public health needs of your communities.

Adaptive leadership is a leadership style that emphasizes the ability of a leader to position their organization's teams to adapt and respond to the complex and rapidly changing challenges in today's organizations and environments.[6,7] The central premise of adaptive leadership is that leaders need to be able to navigate through uncertain and dynamic situations, mobilize their teams to tackle tough problems, and facilitate organizational change in rapidly changing environments. Adaptive leadership differs from technical leadership. Technical leadership requires the application of expertise and experience to solve problems. Adaptive leadership involves skills such as observing and interpreting patterns, challenging the status quo, experimenting with new approaches, and mobilizing teams to face challenges collaboratively.

In public health agencies, the concept of adaptive strategy recognizes that the public health and health care landscape is dynamic and unpredictable. Likewise, strategic thinking equips the organization with the ability to adapt and evolve as circumstances change. Key characteristics of an adaptive strategy include (1) flexibility, (2) rapid decision-making, (3) open communication, (4) a learning focus, (5) environmental scanning and scenario planning, and (6) adaptable resource allocation.

Flexibility

The concept of adaptive strategy emphasizes the importance of being able to change an organization's course quickly. It involves creating structures and processes that allow an organization to shift resources, priorities, and strategic goals when necessary to address emerging issues and trends. While it is difficult to achieve flexibility in large government bureaucracies, it is possible. The experience of COVID showed just how important flexibility is to effective public health practice even when working within seemingly rigid organizations. During COVID, leaders quickly adapted organizational structures and staff duties in response to new demands.

Rapid Decision-Making

Adaptive strategies require leaders to quickly respond to new opportunities and challenges. To accomplish rapid decision-making, strategic goals and overall priorities must be clear to everyone in the organization so that when they are faced with the need to make a quick decision, they can rapidly align decision-making with their organization's strategy.

Open Communication

The adaptive strategy concept requires that communication channels are kept open and are transparent across the organization. Open communication allows for the honest sharing of barriers to progress on reaching organizational goals and opportunities to improve. Open communication ensures that information flows freely between teams and the entire organization is aware of challenges, changes, and new directions.

A Learning Focus

The concept of adaptive strategy promotes a culture of learning and experimentation. Organizations that embrace adaptive strategy encourage employees to acquire new skills and knowledge, foster flexibility and adaptability, and create learning organizations willing to support staff innovation with robust quality improvement and quality assurance processes.[8]

Environmental Scanning and Scenario Planning

The adaptive strategy concept involves monitoring the external environment to identify trends, shifts, and emerging technologies. This helps an organization anticipate changes and respond proactively to a changing horizon or new opportunities. Similarly, organizations using adaptive strategies often engage in scenario planning, in which staff create multiple potential future scenarios and develop strategies to address each one.

Adaptable Resource Allocation

Using the adaptive strategy concept requires organizations to adjust their allocation of resources to meet changing circumstances. Flexible resource allocation ensures that organizational resources can quickly be redirected to capitalize on emerging opportunities or address unanticipated challenges. Flexibility in resource allocation proved to be a significant barrier to using adaptive strategies in public health agencies during COVID. Rigid federal funding requirements about staff time allocations and agency procurement rules made it challenging for leaders to quickly move personnel and supplies within public health agencies to support new demands. As a result, it was extremely difficult for staff to quickly expand their work to support the demand for services such as contract tracing and vaccination programs.

Adaptive leadership emphasizes the importance of aligning leadership behavior with strategic goals. Adaptive leaders play a critical role in guiding organizations through change.[6,7] Strategic thinking includes analyzing how an organization must adapt and change in response to emerging and potential challenges and opportunities. As such, it is critical for strategic thinkers to consider enhancing their adaptive leadership competency and their ability to develop adaptive strategies.

WHY IS STRATEGIC THINKING IMPORTANT TO PUBLIC HEALTH?

Strategic thinking is imperative in the field of public health due to the complex and dynamic nature of public health challenges and the need to effectively prioritize resource allocation to improve population health and well-being. Public health priorities, such as controlling disease outbreaks, achieving racial equity in health outcomes, and addressing environmental health threats are multifaceted and require comprehensive strategies to be addressed effectively. Strategic thinking helps public health professionals analyze and understand the complexities of these challenges and supports the development of effective interventions to address them.

Another advantage of strategic thinking is that it supports innovation by encouraging individuals to explore new possibilities. This helps organizations stay ahead of and adapt to change as they contemplate alternative futures. Just like any private industry corporation or nonprofit organization, governmental public health agencies have to position themselves strategically and compete to stay relevant to receive funding and support from policymakers and to best serve the public. By considering strategic themes and trends, agencies can imagine alternative futures and remain relevant.

In 2017, my colleague Brian Castrucci and I developed five strategic moves for governmental public health agencies (Figure 2-1).[9] These five moves are prompts that public health leaders can use to explore their agencies' roles and priorities in increasingly complex futures. The five strategic moves are as follows: (1) from programs to populations, (2) from clinic to community, (3) from patients to policies, (4) from small to big data, and (5) from regionalization to rationalization.[9]

1. From programs to populations: This strategic move is about how leaders can use strategic thinking to coordinate agency activities across disparate public health activities. Given the numerous programs and often overlapping populations served by public

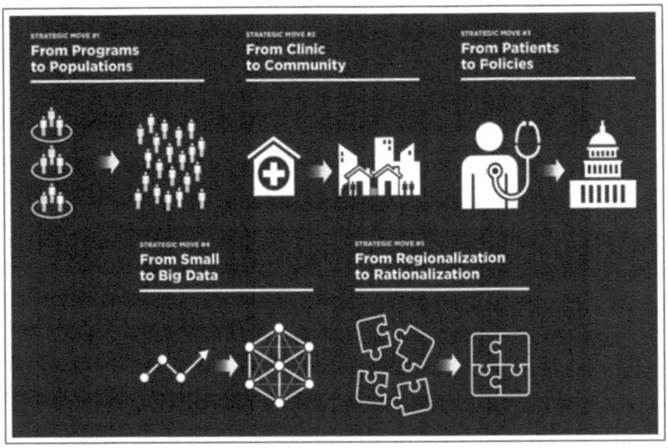

Source: Fraser.[9] Reprinted with permission of Wolters Kluwer Health, Inc.

Figure 2-1. Five Strategic Moves for Public Health

health agencies, strategic thinking can help governmental public health agencies position themselves to consider the interactions that community members may have with various parts of their agencies, and the funding sources that are available to meet shared population health goals.

2. From clinic to community: This strategic move pushes leaders to think about the ongoing transformation in many public health agencies where traditional clinical services, such as providing primary care for uninsured residents, have been moved out of the agency and taken on by other healthcare partners.[9] In these cases, the public health agency's role may be implementing community- and jurisdiction-wide population health improvement activities rather than providing individual-level clinical services. Strategic thinking in this area includes asking what is the role of governmental public health agencies in providing clinical services to individuals as more health systems consolidate and move toward upstream disease prevention work. If more individuals have access to care through community health center expansion and the Affordable Care Act, where should public health agencies focus their work?
3. From patients to policies: This strategic move asks leaders to consider the breadth of a public health agency's impact. Given that public health policies can have a much larger impact on a population's health than individual-level, client-focused interventions, what is the public health agency's role in both advancing policies that protect and improve health and providing patient-level services? How can public health agencies maximize health improvement through policies that make the healthy choice the default or easy choice, or otherwise guide behavior toward better health outcomes?
4. From small to big data: With the rapid development of new technologies such as app-based tools for telehealth consultation, the use of AI in health care and public health,

and federal data-sharing standards for the exchange of data between various health-related entities, how should public health agencies position themselves to integrate with other entities and protect patient privacy and confidentiality? This prompt asks leaders to focus their strategic thinking on data systems improvements within public health agencies and their connections to healthcare and other governmental health agencies. Do legacy disease surveillance and reporting systems have a role in the future, and if not, what are the alternatives? How could agencies position themselves to modernize their enterprise data infrastructure, given new initiatives?

5. From regionalization to rationalization: This prompt asks leaders to consider what foundational public health capabilities should be available in every health agency, and how to align limited resources to achieve economies of scale across various public health jurisdictions. With new federal investments in state and local public health infrastructure and opportunities to build public health capabilities and capacities nationwide, does it make sense to consider pooling resources and consolidating smaller health agencies to reach economies of scale and standardize which public health services are available in every community? What does a rationally distributed public health capacity look like in states with hundreds of local governments, each of which supports a local public health department or board of health? How should state and local health officials engage strategically in planning for more rational distribution of public health services in their jurisdictions?

Discussions of these five strategic moves and the changes they may require can help spur strategic thinking. These moves, and the questions they raise for public health leaders, support opportunities to think about potential futures for their agencies as their communities' chief health strategists. While not the only strategic moves that health agencies may consider, these prompts represent some of the biggest strategic challenges facing governmental public health agencies today.

Strategic thinking in public health helps to support the alignment of very different programs within a single agency. It also connects widely dissimilar health agency programs such as shellfish fishery inspection, breastfeeding promotion, and HIV prevention, and shows how these programs fit together by creating a comprehensive set of public health goals. Strategic thinking and the agency's strategic plan are the blueprints that leaders can use to align disparate services, develop cohesive linkages across the organization's programs, and position the organization to address critical public health issues.

STRATEGIC THINKING AND STRATEGIC PLANNING

Strategic thinking involves individuals working together to analyze complex problems, assessing their organizational environment, and developing creative and innovative solutions to achieve long-term strategic goals and objectives. Strategic thinking is different from tactical thinking, which focuses on short-term goals and immediate actions. Strategic thinking requires a broad perspective and understanding of the organization's strengths, weaknesses, opportunities, and threats.

Strategic planning involves making strategic thinking real in an organization and moving from thinking to tactics by developing action plans to achieve goals and objectives. As Bryson notes, strategic planning is "a disciplined effort to produce fundamental decisions and actions that shape and guide what an organization is, what it does, and why it does it."[10(p2)] Importantly, strategic thinking should also stress what an organization is not going to do, especially if another agency can do the same thing and do it faster, better, or cheaper.

The outcome of strategic planning is a set of tactics to help operationalize strategic thinking. The combination of both strategic thinking and strategic planning results in the organization's strategic plan: a set of goals, objectives, tactics, and measures that lays out the organization's direction for a set period of time. Unfortunately, many strategic plans are not strategic, despite being called such by those who developed them. A list of aspirations is not strategic. Such a list may be encouraging and inspirational, but strategic goals and priorities must be firmly rooted in the reality of an agency's resources and the trade-offs leaders are willing to make.

STEPS IN THE STRATEGIC PLANNING PROCESS

There are many different approaches that organizations can take to develop their strategic plans. While there is no single best approach to strategic planning, most strategic planning processes share several steps. These include establishing or affirming the agency's mission, vision, and values, conducting situational analyses and assessments of the organization's internal and external environments, setting long-term goals and objectives, developing tactical work plans, and monitoring and evaluating progress (for a complete list of terminology used in strategic planning processes, see Appendix A).

Establishing Mission, Vision, and Values Statements

In this step, agency leaders and staff ask and answer questions about what the organization wants to see in the world, why the agency exists, and how it will behave in working to realize its vision. Mission and vision statements should be clear and concise and describe the organization's overall purpose (mission) and its ideal future (vision). Values statements help guide organizational behavior by stating how staff will accomplish their work and setting expectations for how organizational members will interact with each other and with partners and stakeholders. In many instances, the agency's mission, vision, and values will stay the same across multiple organizational strategic plans. However, it is important to review these statements and affirm their relevance as part of any strategic planning process.

Conducting Situational Analyses and Assessments

In this step, organizations conduct thorough analyses of their current organizational position and identify the opportunities and challenges that they face in their external environment. Tools to help with these assessments, such as a strengths, weaknesses, opportunities, and threats (SWOT) analysis or strategic foresight are described in the following section.

Setting Goals and Objectives

This step involves developing goals and objectives that are specific, measurable, achievable, relevant, and time bound (or SMART) and that also describe the organizational efforts needed to carry out the agency's mission and realize its vision.[10] Examples of strategic goals, objectives, and tactics are provided in Appendix A.

Developing Tactical Work Plans

In this step, staff develop tactical work plans to achieve their goals and objectives. This includes developing timelines and identifying the resources needed. Tactical workplans can also be used to develop individual staff performance plans and align staff workplans.

Monitoring and Evaluating Progress

A key task of organizational management teams is to monitor and evaluate the agency's progress toward meeting stated goals and objectives and adjust work as needed. Staff should also report on progress to stakeholders and leaders responsible for overseeing the strategic plan. In organizations with a board of directors, the board generally provides oversight of strategic plan implementation to ensure that its goals and priorities are accomplished by the professional staff of an organization. In government, the legislature may serve this role and may receive periodic updates on the public health agency's progress toward reaching priorities and goals.

Strategic planning is an essential tool for organizational success, particularly in the face of uncertainty and change. By setting clear goals and objectives and developing tactical plans to achieve them, organizations can better adapt to changing circumstances and stay relevant in their environment. A strategic planning process and the development of a strategic plan are also critical requirements for public health agencies to meet voluntary public health accreditation standards.

STRATEGIC PLANNING AS A ROAD TRIP

There are many analogies that can be used to make the process more familiar to individuals starting out on their strategic planning journey. I use the metaphor of a road trip, or similar driving adventure. When I was a kid, our family used get in the car on Sunday afternoons and just go for a drive. Squashed in the back seat with my siblings, we had no idea where we were headed or what we were going to be doing during the ride. Neither did my parents, who would pick a place, change directions on the way, and find interesting antique shops and oddities along the route that would become our waypoints. We never knew what we would find or where we would stop until the spirit moved the driver to pull over and explore. It was certainly entertaining and kept us all busy on a Sunday afternoon. But it was also the exact opposite of strategic: it was spontaneous and reactive.

By contrast, strategic planning is about picking a destination or goal. In this road trip analogy, strategic goals would be the destination of our journey or our end point. Our strategic plan would be our map: it would be clear where we were headed and everyone in the car would know that from the outset. While it may lack the spontaneity of an unplanned adventure, having a destination would be far more efficient than just driving around on a random weekend jaunt. Knowing our goal, we could all prepare for our trip. We would know how long we would be gone, what snacks to pack, and whether we would need a bathing suit or a sweater. Clarity of goals and objectives, that is, knowing where you are going and how you are going to get there, allows everyone in an organization to "get on the same page" when it comes to the journey.

If our drive's destination is our goal, our waypoints along the route are our objectives. One objective may be to stop and get breakfast, then perhaps we would visit a sight we had never seen before or stop in at a friend's place. Objectives are our drive's stops, and meeting them allows us track our progress. Tactics would be how we drive, including the car we take, our speed, the directions we would be heading, our timing, and the fuel needed to reach our goal. Tactics and objectives contribute to our goal and clarify the waypoints, processes, and resources needed to get to our destination. While simple, I find this analogy helpful in making the components of a strategic plan clear.

STRATEGIC THINKING AND PLANNING TOOLS

There are several tools that can be used to help people engage in strategic thinking and support an organization's strategic planning process. These tools include assessments that can evaluate an organization's current efforts and allow it to develop new goals given potential futures. While the strategic planning process involves specific steps, and planning requires assigning tasks and timelines to various tactics, it is important to remember that strategic planning, just like strategic thinking, is not linear or fixed.[11] As you develop and implement your strategic plan, your environment may change and your plan must adapt to new factors, including both threats and opportunities in your environment. Zweifel and Borey address this issue:

> [T]he world has changed. Speed, globalization, the Internet and virtual teams, new technologies, democratization and flatter hierarchies, empowerment and the growing importance of the knowledge worker, and increasing complexity have combined to change fundamentally how companies must do business. In a complex, dynamic, and uncertain world, traditional planning methods are non-starters.[11(p22)]

Whenever you are developing strategies and conducting strategic planning, keep in mind that you may need to adapt to rapid change as you implement your plan's goals and objectives over time. It is also important to remember that it is the act of planning and strategic thinking, not the plan document itself, that is more valuable to the organization.

Strategy implementation is where many organizations fall short. Far too often, beautifully developed strategic plans that are the result of hours or days of staff time and partner and stakeholder input are left on a shelf to collect dust because no implementation plan was developed. It is imperative that organizations think carefully about strategic plan implementation, not just strategic planning. This includes being realistic about achievable objectives in pursuit of strategic goals, having honest conversations about the resources that the agency has, and identifying what new resources will be needed to carry out its work.

Major tasks of organizational leadership are as follows: ensure that everyone in the organization knows their role in moving the strategic plan forward through constant communication about mission, vision, values, and goals, monitor progress against key metrics, and ensure that teams have the resources needed to accomplish their work. As Bregman states, strategic plan execution and implementation is often a people problem,[12] due to many of the barriers cited by Horwath[1] in his research that was summarized earlier in this chapter. If no one in the agency is held accountable for reaching strategic goals, or no one understands their part in the execution or implementation of the strategic plan, progress on the plan's priorities will stall. Successful management includes identifying, accelerating, and celebrating enablers of progress and resolving barriers to successful plan implementation with staff teams.

One way to support staff implementation of a strategic plan, and to help support strategic thinking, is to include staff in the strategic planning process. Teams can then use planning tools to assess organizational competencies and develop their plans. Several of these tools are described in the following section.

Ask Strategic Questions

Asking strategic questions is essential for an organization to develop a clear vision, set meaningful goals, and create a plan for achieving them. Some of these questions include the following:

- What is our current state, and do our priorities support our organization's vision and mission? Or, more simply put, where are we now?
- What are the emerging trends and opportunities in public health and how can we address them? That is, what is happening around us and how are we responding to and adapting to it?
- What are our core competencies, and how can we leverage them to advance our organizational strategy? What are we good at that makes us successful and unique?
- What are some ways that we can improve our organizational culture, and create or sustain an environment that fosters innovation and collaboration?
- How do we measure progress towards our strategic goals and adjust our plans as needed?

If you started to answer the questions in the previous list as you were reading them, you now have a sense of the rich conversations about strategy that will ensue. The questions that follow are similar to the previous questions, but are adapted for public health agency strategy development:

- What are the key public health issues in our community or region? What are the prevalent diseases, health disparities, and social determinants of health that need to be addressed? What measures can we take to reduce health disparities among different demographic groups? How can we promote health equity?
- How can we effectively engage the community in our public health efforts? What strategies can we use to involve community members and other organizations in informing and shaping public health initiatives and strategic goals? How can we build trust and collaboration within the various communities we serve to help support our objectives?
- What are our overarching public health goals and objectives? What are the long-term health outcomes we want to achieve for the population we serve? How can we promote overall health and well-being?
- What resources are available, and what resources are needed, to accomplish our objectives? What funding, personnel, and infrastructure are required to support existing and future public health programs and interventions? How can we secure additional resources if necessary?
- What evidence-based practices and interventions do we need to implement to reach our public health goals? What research and data inform our strategy development? How can we adapt evidence-based practices to our specific community or population?
- What are the legal and ethical considerations involved in our work? How do ethical principles and legal regulations and requirements impact organizational decision-making and strategy setting?
- What are the collaborations we want to develop and/or sustain with other stakeholders? How can public health agencies work with healthcare providers, local governments, schools, and nonprofit organizations to achieve common health goals?

Box 2-1. Sample PEST Analysis Questions for a Public Health Agency

Political Factors	Economic Factors
• Government regulations and policies: What is the impact of government policies such as funding, vaccination mandates, or disease control measures on public health? • Political stability: How will changes in government leadership or political stability affect public health initiatives and funding? • Public health advocacy: What is the level of political support for public health programs and initiatives, including lobbying efforts by advocacy groups?	• Funding: What is the allocation of funds for public health programs and what is our assessment of the impact of budget changes in the next year? • Economic conditions: What is the state of the economy, such as unemployment rates, income levels, and access to services, and what is its influence on the public's health? • Labor market: What employment trends are impacting our workforce? What do we need to do to compete for talent?
Social Factors	**Technological Factors**
• Demographics: What are the demographic characteristics of the populations served by our agency? • Health behaviors: What are public attitudes and behaviors related to health, including smoking, diet, exercise, and vaccination compliance? • Cultural factors: What cultural beliefs, norms, and practices may impact public health campaigns and interventions in our jurisdiction?	• Advances in technology: What is the impact of technologies, such as telemedicine, electronic health records, AI, and new diagnostic tools, on public health service delivery? • Data collection and analysis: What is our current and future ability to collect and analyze health data to inform decision-making and policy development? What are barriers to data sharing? • Communication technology: What technology can we use to disseminate evidence-based health information and engage with the public?

Note: AI = artificial intelligence; PEST = political, economic, social, and technological factors.

Discussions of these questions set the stage for strategy development while also getting you to start thinking about your organization's challenges and how to position it to address them. These questions also support strategic thinking about partnerships, collaboration, and other organizations that may share strategic goals and help accomplish shared strategic objectives.

PEST Analysis

In addition to asking strategic questions and using the answers to draft organizational strategy, you can also undertake a series of structured exercises and assessments to craft your priorities and goals. PEST stands for political, economic, social, and technological factors, and a PEST analysis is an assessment that helps organizations understand the external factors that may impact their work (Box 2-1). A PEST analysis can help organizations identify potential opportunities and threats in the external environment.

Using a PEST analysis, your team can identify key political, economic, social, and technological factors that will influence the environment in which it crafts organizational strategy. When used in conjunction with other strategic thinking tools, such as a SWOT analysis, a PEST analysis can lead to a comprehensive understanding of your agency's opportunities and potential barriers to progress.

One variation on the PEST analysis is the PESTLE analysis, which includes political, economic, social, and technological factors, as well as legal and environmental factors that may influence the organization's positioning. The PESTLE framework was developed by the Public Health Foundation. It sorts factors by whether or not the organization has direct control of the factor (such as by developing partnerships with key stakeholders in the faith community), whether the organization has the ability to influence the factor (such as by advocating at the state legislature for a particular policy), and what factors might be outside of the organization's influence and control entirely (such as economic indicators).[13] The PESTLE framework provides a look at the agency's operational context that is even more comprehensive than a PEST analysis.

SWOT Analysis

A SWOT (strengths, weaknesses, opportunities, and threats) analysis is a common tool used in strategic planning processes. Strengths are internal organizational assets, such as a talented and skilled workforce, efficient processes, or influence. Weaknesses are internal factors that the organization needs to improve, such as the use of outdated technology systems or limited financial resources. Opportunities are external factors that the organization can leverage to its advantage, such as new grant programs, changes in public health regulations, or new technologies. Threats are external factors that could negatively impact the organization, such as increased distrust of public health officials, economic downturns, or environmental concerns such as more extreme weather events.

A SWOT analysis includes meetings of agency staff, partner groups, stakeholders, and community members. The planning team identifies and discusses each of the four parts of the SWOT (Box 2-2), using data and evidence to support their conclusions. The discussion can help organizations identify key areas of focus for strategic planning and develop action plans to address the identified strengths, weaknesses, opportunities, and threats.

SWOT participants then discuss the impact of each of the items in the SWOT analysis and the implications for how to position the agency. This leads to the development of goals and priorities that the agency could pursue as it responds to external opportunities and threats and addresses internal weaknesses, while leveraging its strengths. Opportunities and strengths can provide support for innovation and sustain success as the organization moves forward. Weaknesses and threats are areas to address as strategy is developed and implemented.

Box 2-2. Sample SWOT Analysis for a Public Health Agency

Strengths	Weaknesses
• Qualified staff: We have a team of highly skilled and experienced public health professionals. • Strong community partnerships: We have established and strong partnerships with local healthcare providers, community organizations, and other government agencies. • Effective disease surveillance system: There is a robust disease surveillance system in place, enabling early detection and response to outbreaks. • Effective communication channels: Staff are experts in communication, utilizing various social media channels to support public health efforts. • Grant funding: We secure consistent grant funding, allowing us to support a wide range of public health programs and initiatives.	• Limited resources: We face resource constraints, particularly in terms of funding and staffing, which can hinder progress. • Bureaucratic processes: Complex procedures and slow decision-making can sometimes impede our ability to respond swiftly to emerging public health threats. • Data management challenges: We have challenges managing data in one system and then sharing data among different divisions within the agency that use different systems. • Workforce retention: A high turnover rate among staff has led to a loss of institutional knowledge and disruption in the continuity of programs (largely due to low salaries and staff retirements).
Opportunities	**Threats**
• Technology: There are opportunities to use AI and data analytics to enhance the agency's data collection, analysis, and response capabilities. • Public health education initiatives: The growing awareness of the importance of public health presents an opportunity to expand public health education campaigns. • Policy advocacy: We can actively engage in policy advocacy to influence legislation that supports public health goals and secures additional funding. • Pandemic preparedness/infrastructure: Recent global health crises have highlighted the need for improved pandemic preparedness, creating opportunities to strengthen response capabilities and infrastructure.	• Budget cuts: Economic downturns and shifts in government priorities may lead to reduced funding for public health programs and services. • Emerging diseases: The constant threat of new and emerging diseases strains the agency's resources; a need for surge capacity remains. • Health disparities: Ongoing health disparities within the community pose challenges to achieving equitable public health outcomes. • Anti-vaccination policy: Growing anti-vaccine sentiment threatens public health progress. • Trust in government: Declining trust in government may erode support for public health agencies and our programs.

Note: AI = artificial intelligence; SWOT = strengths, weaknesses, opportunities and threats.

Scenario Planning

Scenario planning is a tool that organizations can use to consider potential futures and develop strategies that anticipate them. Scenario planning also helps organizations plan for uncertainty as scenarios can be developed that include how uncertainty may play out over time. It involves depicting potential future realities and discussing their impact on public health agency strategy and operations. Agency staff can develop potential scenarios about how the future may unfold and use these scenarios to help clarify how envisioned trends and changes may impact strategy. While the futures developed are fictional, they help an agency anticipate potentially real changes and identify actual threats and opportunities more easily.

In 2017, the Association of State and Territorial Health Officials (ASTHO) used scenario planning to anticipate potential futures for public health. The Public Health 2035 scenarios helped ASTHO assess strategic opportunities in the future and evaluate how the association should prepare to support health agencies.[14] Three scenarios were developed by the ASTHO staff and board of directors and the staff of the Institute for Alternative Futures. Each scenario represents a potential future to which public health agencies and ASTHO would have to respond in the year 2035.

Scenario 1: Improved Health, but Disparities Persist

Amid recurring political, fiscal, and health challenges, public health agencies and health care slowly advance their capabilities. Many use automation and advanced analytics to improve services and community and population health. However, environmental trends and other crises increasingly challenge the health and well-being of the nation, and there is little progress in improving the social determinants of health. Great variations in technological capabilities, funding, and approaches to prevention—along with a continuous rise in health care costs—significantly limit public health gains.

Scenario 2: Overwhelmed, Under-Resourced

Public health crises grow worse and more frequent, largely due to environmental trends. Funding cuts, a hostile political context, and information wars undermine the role and effectiveness of public health agencies. Failures cement a public perception of government agencies as ineffective "nanny state" bureaucratic strongholds. Private sector initiatives produce significant innovations for health and wellness, but these primarily benefit middle-class and affluent groups. Technological, economic, educational, and health disparities grow, and public health institutions have limited power to change this trend.

Scenario 3: Optimal Health for All

National and local economies gradually grow, and new advances help households sustain themselves and improve health and well-being. Changes in values and demographics lead to health considerations in all policymaking and support for inclusion, fairness, and equal opportunity for all. Public health agencies use advanced analytics, gamification, and diverse partnerships to identify problems and opportunities and catalyze and incentivize action to improve community health. While some disparities persist, the vast majority of

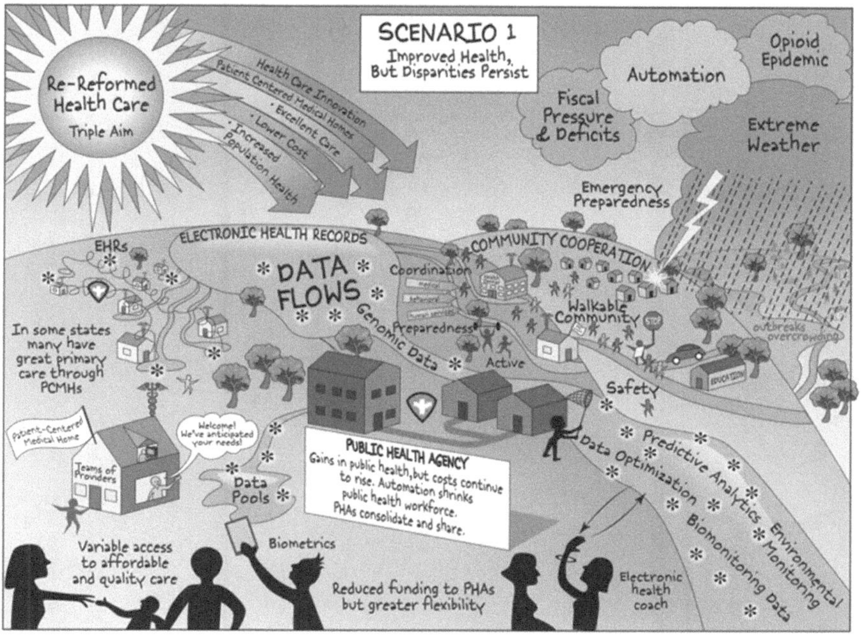

Source: Institute for Alternative Futures and ASTHO.[14] Reprinted with permission of ASTHO.

Figure 2-2. Scenario 1: Improved Health, But Disparities Persist

US residents have greater opportunities for good health through quality improvements in housing, economic opportunity, education, and other social determinants of health.[1(p4)]

Images depicting each scenario were developed by Institute for Alternative Futures illustrators to help the staff and board envision these potential futures more clearly (Figures 2-2, 2-3 and 2-4).[14] Within each image are factors that characterize the potential future and the trends that health officials would need to consider as they lead their agencies forward. Elements of all three scenarios have become reality since they were developed, because no single scenario could accurately predict the future. Discussions of these three scenarios, even with the long-term horizon of the year 2035, helped ASTHO leadership develop strategies and goals that could adapt to these potential future environments. Similar scenario planning for your organization's potential futures may be valuable for your planning and strategy development.

Strategic Foresight

Strategic foresight is the process of systematically exploring future developments that may impact an organization's work and crafting strategies to respond to them. Strategic foresight uses structured approaches to anticipate trends in technological, demographic,

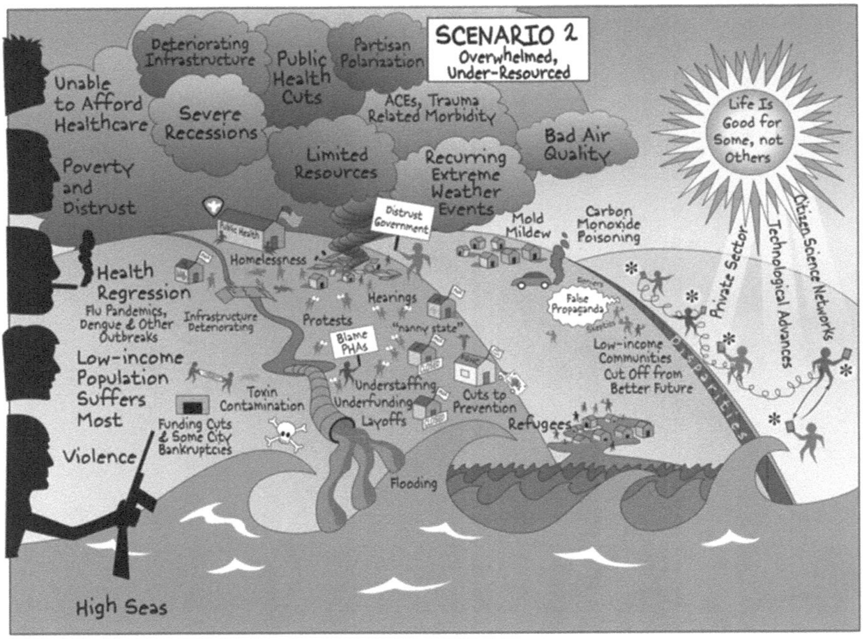

Source: Institute for Alternative Futures and ASTHO.[14] Reprinted with permission of ASTHO.

Figure 2-3. Scenario 2: Overwhelmed, Under-Resourced

political, or economic environments that may impact an organization. The information gathered through strategic foresight is used to inform an organization's strategic planning process, allowing staff to develop strategies that are proactive and future oriented. An organization may use strategic foresight to identify new programs and services in a growing segment of the population; for example, given the growing population of older Americans, age-friendly public health programs might be identified. Foresight work may also ask public health agencies to consider the potential for self-driving cars to help expand access to public health and health care services in a community.

The process of strategic foresight can involve both internal and external stakeholders, such as employees, stakeholders, community members, and industry experts. As part of the foresight process, it is important to gather information from sectors outside your own and ask how trends in other sectors may impact your sector. For example, foresight work specific to public health may want to look to education, housing, economic development, technology, and transportation to see which developments in these sectors might influence the public health sector. Key to strategic foresight is the collection of information on potential signals in the environment that may evolve into significant issues. These signals are found by scanning different areas for new trends that could affect both the organization and the community it serves. There are several future trends and emerging

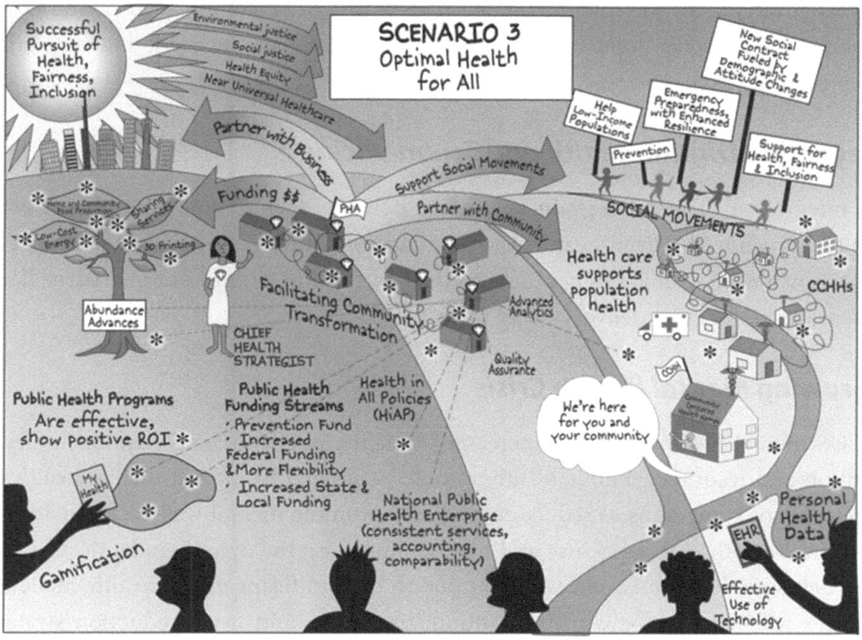

Source: Institute for Alternative Futures and ASTHO.[14] Reprinted with permission of ASTHO.

Figure 2-4. Scenario 3: Optimal Health for All

issues that are likely to have a significant impact on public health agencies. Here are some strategic foresight examples for growing trends that you can use to think about how to strategically position your work.

Increasing Global Health Threats

Public health agencies will need to continuously adapt to new and evolving global health threats, such as pandemics (e.g., COVID), emerging infectious diseases, and antimicrobial resistance. Preparedness, rapid response, and international collaboration will be key focus areas. Local and state health departments will need to closely collaborate with federal officials to monitor disease trends and understand travel and migration patterns that might impact their jurisdictions.

Addressing Racial Equity, Health Equity, and Social Determinants of Health

There is growing recognition of the importance of addressing racial equity and health equity to improve health. Public health agencies will need to continue to advance work that promotes racial equity and health equity and to work across program areas to support equity in the jurisdictions they serve. This will be complicated by the growth of increasingly diverse populations and pushback against equity work and community power building in many areas.

Integrating Digital Health and Telemedicine

The integration of technology in healthcare delivery, including telemedicine, remote monitoring, and AI-driven health data analytics will continue to evolve. Public health agencies will need to adapt to new data sources and digital tools to improve surveillance, prevention, and service delivery using these tools.

A Growing Mental Health Crisis

The US mental health crisis has increased since the pandemic and requires increased attention and resources. Public health agencies will need to expand mental health services, sponsor campaigns to reduce stigma, and promote mental well-being in addition to physical health. Substance use and misuse, including the opioid epidemic, as well as other behavioral health issues, will continue to be significant public health challenges. Agencies will need to focus on prevention, treatment, and harm reduction strategies while positioning themselves alongside other agencies that provide services to address mental health needs in their jurisdictions.

Mistrust of Government

Over the last several years, there has been a trend toward increasing mistrust of government, and by extension, public health agencies. This trend has been fueled by various factors, including the spread of misinformation and conspiracy theories, skepticism about the handling of public health crises, and a general erosion of trust in government institutions nationwide. The COVID pandemic exacerbated these issues, with public health guidelines and vaccination efforts often becoming politicized and polarized. To address this growing mistrust, there is a pressing need for transparent and effective communication from government agencies and focused, collaborative efforts to rebuild trust in government.

An Aging Population

As the population ages, public health agencies will need to address the public health and health care needs of older adults. These include not only chronic disease management and caregiving support but also social connectedness and addressing the isolation that many seniors experience. This is an area that is not traditionally part of public health agency portfolios, but it will become increasingly important as the aging population grows in the United States.

Addressing the Health Impacts of Climate Change

Public health agencies play a role in addressing the health impacts of climate change. These include the impact of extreme weather events, worsening air and water quality, and the spread of vector-borne diseases. Addressing these health impacts will be complicated by the efforts of some members of the community who deny that climate change exists and oppose taking actions that reduce greenhouse gas emissions.

ASTHO Scan Priorities

ASTHO compiles an annual scan of priority issues for state and territorial public health agencies. These scans help health officials prepare for trends that may need to be addressed by their health agencies. The ASTHO scans are developed using qualitative and quantitative methods to identify state health agency priorities and issues of concern for health officials. ASTHO then uses these priorities to anticipate technical assistance and capacity-building requests to inform its advocacy efforts and ensure that its programming and policy capacity can address the priorities that are relevant to its members.

In 2023, ASTHO identified five key priorities as part of its environmental scanning activities[15]:

1. Maternal, child, and family health, including youth and adolescent physical and mental well-being, early childhood development and health promotion, prenatal and perinatal care, and maternal and infant mortality.
2. Behavioral health and substance use, including mental health, suicide prevention, substance misuse prevention, substance use harm reduction, treatment and recovery services, and opioid use.
3. Access to and linkage with health care, including primary and preventive care, health insurance coverage and care affordability, economic barriers to healthcare access, quality of care, inequities in healthcare outcomes, and coordination and continuity of care.
4. Communicable disease control, including immunization and vaccination, sexually transmitted infections and diseases, HIV/AIDS, and building capacity for communicable disease laboratory testing and monitoring.
5. Chronic disease prevention, including nutrition, physical activity and other modifiable personal health behaviors, tobacco and vaping, and healthy weight/obesity prevention.

These ASTHO scan priorities can be used to inform strategic foresight efforts by revealing current and emerging public health trends. For example, as rates of chronic disease continue to increase, agencies can ask which activities, programs, and policies public health leaders should develop or sustain to position their organizations to more effectively promote chronic disease prevention. Using these priorities and discussing their implications as trends change are ways to help an organization plan for an uncertain future.

Strategic Maps

Strategic maps, also known as strategy maps or balanced scorecards, are tools used to communicate an organization's strategy and objectives.[16,17] A strategic map is usually presented in a grid or diagram format and typically includes four key perspectives, as follows: (1) financial, (2) customer, (3) internal processes, and (4) learning and growth.[17]

Financial Perspective

The financial perspective highlights the financial goals and objectives of the organization, such as revenue growth, cost reduction, and profitability. In governmental public health this may include grant revenue growth and grant spend-down rates, rather than private sector indicators such as profitability.

Customer or Community Perspective

The customer or community perspective focuses on the needs and preferences of the individuals and communities that interact with the organization and how these needs can be met. This perspective may include metrics such as customer satisfaction, retention, or loyalty. In public health agencies, customers are usually the individuals and the population served by the agency.

Internal Processes Perspective

The internal processes perspective focuses on key business processes and activities that support the organization's objectives. Metrics such as process efficiency, quality, and innovation help measure the performance of internal processes. In public health agencies, this may include time to hire or workforce retention rates, time to procure goods and services, or time for payment of contracts.

Learning and Growth Perspective

The learning and growth perspective focuses on the organization's human resources, including employee skills and knowledge, as well as its organizational culture. This perspective may include metrics such as employee satisfaction, training and development completion, or knowledge sharing across the organization.

Strategic maps are typically developed by teams of stakeholders, including leaders, employees, and customers or community members, and are designed to provide concise overviews of organizational strategy and objectives. A strategic map can help to align stakeholders around a common vision and provide a framework for monitoring progress and adjusting as needed. A sample strategic map for a public health agency, using the balanced scorecard framework, is depicted in Box 2-3. In addition to the four typical

Box 2-3. Sample Strategic Map Using the Balanced Scorecard Framework for a Public Health Agency

Financial Perspective	Customer/Community Perspective
Objective: Ensure financial sustainability and efficient resource allocation. *Measures:* • Total budget allocation and utilization. • Diversity of grants and funding sources. • Cost per public health program or service. • Revenue generated from fees.	*Objective:* Deliver high-quality public health services and meet community needs. *Measures:* • Patient satisfaction. • Access to healthcare services. • Timeliness of services provided. • Community health needs assessment completed.
Internal Process Perspective	**Learning and Growth Perspective**
Objective: Streamline and improve internal processes to enhance service delivery. *Measures:* • Process efficiency metrics (e.g., wait times, appointment scheduling). • Compliance with standards and regulations. • Program evaluation and quality improvement efforts. • Employee satisfaction and retention.	*Objective:* Invest in workforce development, innovation, and technology. *Measures:* • Staff training and development programs. • Employee skills and competencies. • Adoption of new IT systems. • Innovation and research initiatives.
Public Health Outcomes Perspective	**Stakeholder and Partner Perspective**
Objective: Achieve positive health outcomes and improve the overall health of the community. *Measures:* • Disease prevention and control measures (e.g., vaccination rates, disease surveillance rates). • Reductions in health disparities by race. • Health outcomes (e.g., life expectancy, disease prevalence).	*Objective:* Foster strong relationships with stakeholders and partners. *Measures:* • Stakeholder satisfaction and engagement. • Collaborative projects and partnerships. • Compliance with reporting requirements. • Community involvement and public awareness.

Note: IT = information technology.

perspectives (financial, internal process, customer/community, learning and growth), two additional perspectives were added (public health outcomes and stakeholder and partners) for an even richer analysis of agency activities.

This example map may help an agency measure its performance, track progress, and improve public health outcomes. The addition of two perspectives for a public health example demonstrates that these tools are flexible and that you can add and adjust strategic maps depending on your specific needs and organizational capabilities.

There are many tools you can use to help promote strategic thinking and develop strategic plans in your organization. Starting with simple questions about your agency can be helpful as you and your team add dedicated time to think strategically about your work. PEST and SWOT analyses can help you assess internal and external environment issues. Scenario planning and strategic foresight tools can help you identify important trends and reveal early signals of issues that you may need to anticipate as your agency moves its strategy forward. The goal of these tools is to actively and routinely engage your team, stakeholders, and community members in efforts to identify strategic issues and your organization's ability to anticipate and react to them.

IMPLEMENTING STRATEGIC THINKING IN PUBLIC HEALTH

Overcoming barriers to strategic thinking requires a combination of awareness, skill, and practice. Here are some ways that you can make sure you are thinking strategically:

1. Make time for strategic thinking: All staff, but especially leaders, need to prioritize and dedicate sufficient time and resources to strategic thinking. Some colleagues I know add blocks of one to two hours in their weekly schedule to make sure they have time dedicated to strategic thinking and study.
2. Encourage diverse perspectives: Strategic thinkers seek out diverse perspectives and opinions, including those that challenge their own assumptions and beliefs. Questions to ask to make sure you are encouraging diverse perspectives include the following: Who else should I be talking to about this issue? Who that we do not normally include needs to be at the table for our planning discussions, and what might different members of our staff, stakeholder groups, or community think about this issue? How do these perspectives impact our goals and objectives?
3. Encourage horizontal connections between staff: All staff, not just leaders, can break down silos that may limit collaboration and sharing by encouraging cross-functional collaboration and communication. Start by thinking about activities that might be common across your organization, such as addressing health equity, communications, grants management and finance, or policy development. Then, reach out to program leads and technical experts in these areas who might want to collaborate on shared goals.
4. Foster cultures of feedback and accountability: Leaders should create a culture of feedback and accountability, where they are open to receiving feedback and are held accountable for the outcomes of their strategic decisions. Cultivating transparency and communicating about strategy development and implementation are critical to receiving constructive feedback. End meetings by asking for feedback and be sure to share your feedback with others.

5. Embrace change: All staff can promote a culture of innovation and experimentation where new ideas and approaches are encouraged, and failure is seen as an opportunity to learn and improve. Encourage those you work with to learn about change management and engage them in change management efforts. Organizations that manage change well are extremely successful regardless of industry or governance model because they use strategic thinking tools to adapt and evolve.

STRATEGIC PLANNING SHORTFALLS

You would be hard-pressed to find any management or leadership expert who thinks that strategic thinking is unnecessary, but there are many critiques of strategic planning. These critiques focus on strategic plans that are developed without plans to evaluate progress toward goals. Likewise, when done poorly, strategic plans can be too rigid and this rigidity constrains rather than accelerates organizational progress. Rigidity makes it difficult for staff to adapt to changing circumstances and seize new opportunities because of the pressure to execute the already-established plan. Strategic plans are often designed to guide an organization for three to five years, but in today's rapidly changing operating environment, long-term plans can quickly become outdated. In short, strategic planning without ongoing strategic thinking can be problematic. Even after a plan is finalized, adapting, refreshing, and revising it is a constant process.

Some strategic planning processes can be time-consuming and resource intensive, but they do not have to be. Processes that require many staff members to conduct extensive data gathering, analysis, and consultation can become clunky and inefficient. Processes that are not well managed can divert resources and attention away from other, important activities within the organization. Strategic thinkers should actively assess the effort needed to conduct robust planning within the organization and remember that organizational commitment can vary depending on existing staff workloads and perceptions of the utility of the process for their work.

Strategic plans may also create a false sense of security for an organization. Strategic planning may lead some to a perception that an organization has a clear and predictable path to success, as long as they just follow the steps in the plan. However, this may not be the case. External factors can change rapidly and disrupt the best-laid plans. Strategic thinkers know the utility of having a plan but focus more effort on maintaining an ongoing planning process to ensure that their organizations remain strategic. Strategic planning is a valuable tool for organizations, but it is important to be aware of these critiques and to mitigate their impact. By remaining flexible, encouraging diverse perspectives, and regularly reviewing and updating the plan, organizations can use strategic thinking to develop successful strategic plans and adapt to changing circumstances.

REFERENCES

1. Horwath R. *Elevate: The Three Disciplines of Advanced Strategic Thinking.* Wiley; 2014.
2. DeSalvo KB, Wang YC, Harris A, Auerbach J, Koo D, O'Carroll P. Public health 3.0: A call to action for public health to meet the challenges of the 21st century. *Prev Chronic Dis* 2017;14:170017. doi:10.5888/pcd14.170017
3. Ginter PM, Duncan J. Strategic thinking: Rationale, process, and behaviors. In: Helm-Murtagh SC, Erwin P, eds. *Leadership in Practice: Essentials for Public Health and Healthcare Leaders.* Springer Publishing; 2023:55–76.
4. Fraser, MR. Vision, mission, strategy, and culture as core concepts of public health practice. In: Fraser MR, Castrucci BC, eds. *Building Strategic Skills for Better Health: A Primer for Public Health Professionals.* Oxford University Press; 2024:21–37.
5. Tie association calls it quits as trends change. *SouthCoast Today.* June 12, 2008. Accessed January 2, 2024. https://www.southcoasttoday.com/story/news/nation-world/2008/06/12/tie-association-calls-it-quits/52378690007
6. Heifetz RA, Linsky M. *Leadership on the Line: Staying Alive through the Dangers of Leading.* Harvard Business School Press; 2002.
7. Heifetz R, Grashow A, Linsky M. *The Practice of Adaptive Leadership: Tools and Tactics for Changing Your Organization and the World.* Harvard Business Press; 2009.
8. Senge, PM. *The Fifth Discipline: The Art and Practice of the Learning Organization.* Random House; 1990.
9. Fraser MR, Castrucci BC. Beyond the status quo: 5 strategic moves to position state and territorial public health agencies for an uncertain future. *J Public Health Manag Pract.* 2017;23(5):543–551. doi:10.1097/phh.0000000000000634
10. Bryson JM. *Strategic Planning for Public and Nonprofit Organizations: A Guide to Strengthening and Sustaining Organizational Achievement.* Wiley; 2018.
11. Zweifel T, Borey E. *Strategy in Action: Marrying Planning, People, and Performance.* iHorizon; 2013.
12. Bregman P. Execution is a people problem, not a strategy problem. *Harvard Business Review.* January 4, 2017. Accessed January 2, 2024. https://hbr.org/2017/01/execution-is-a-people-problem-not-a-strategy-problem
13. Moran JW, Meadows A. PESTLE Chart. Public Health Foundation. June 2016. Accessed January 2, 2024. https://www.phf.org/resourcestools/Documents/PESTLE_Chart.pdf
14. *Public Health 2035 Scenarios: Divergent Futures.* Institute for Alternative Futures and Association of State and Territorial Health Officials; 2017.
15. Association of State and Territorial Health Officials. 2023 Environmental Scan of Current and Emerging Public Health Priorities. December 4, 2023. Accessed January 2, 2024. https://www.astho.org/topic/research/environmental-scan
16. Kaplan RS, Norton DP. *The Balanced Scorecard: Translating Strategy into Action.* Harvard Business Press; 1996.
17. Kaplan RS, Norton DP. *Strategy Maps: Converting Intangible Assets into Tangible Outcomes.* Harvard Business Review Press; 2004.

3

Conclusion

This primer shares several fundamental concepts and basic tools that you can use to build your competency in the public health skill of systems and strategic thinking. It is my hope that you will use this material to think of new and innovative ways to assess the systems you work within that impact health outcomes in your jurisdictions and your work's strategic directions. As mentioned early in this primer, if there was ever a time for public health professionals to develop and enhance their systems and strategic thinking competency, it is now. Adaptive challenges, not just scientific or technical challenges, abound. The skill of systems and strategic thinking can help you address many of these challenges by assessing the systems in which you are working and using strategic thinking to position your agency and its resources to have the most impact.

As described herein, systems thinking and strategic thinking are important approaches for addressing complex problems and achieving long-term goals, but they do differ in focus and perspective. Systems thinking involves analyzing an entire system, including the inputs, outputs, feedback loops, and other interactions between a system's various parts. It focuses on understanding the underlying structures and dynamics that drive a system's behavior over time. Strategic thinking is primarily focused on setting and achieving long-term organizational goals and objectives. It also involves assessing the organization's internal and external environments and developing strategies and tactics to achieve the desired outcomes.

Systems thinking is essential to effective leadership and success and involves understanding how different components of a system interact with each other and how changes in one area can affect other areas. As described earlier in this primer, systems thinking helps individuals and organizations identify the root causes of public health problems and develop solutions that address underlying causes rather than surface-level problems. Strategic thinking is similarly essential for effective leadership and organizational success because it enables leaders to anticipate and respond to changes in the environment, identify new opportunities, make informed decisions, and promote enterprise-wide versus program-specific connections.

Systems and strategic thinking is a powerful combination that public health professionals can use to fully analyze the contexts in which they are operating, to assess points of intervention for change, and to position their organization's work for potential futures. For example, systems thinking can help identify the underlying drivers of success or failure, while strategic thinking can help identify opportunities for innovation and growth. In sum, the systems and strategic thinking skill is vital to addressing complex problems and achieving long-term goals in public health.

The systems and strategic thinking skill can help you take concrete steps to address the health challenges you face today and in the future. At the core of the systems and strategic thinking skill is the essential need to approach problems and solutions from broad, big-picture perspectives, emphasizing interconnectedness, relationships, patterns, and synergies as well as leverage points for change. Use this material with your colleagues and in your communities to position and align your work to meet shared agency goals. If you want to learn more, there are many additional resources in Appendix B that you can use for further study of systems and strategic thinking.

APPENDICES

Appendix A: Strategic Planning Terminology

There are several terms and phrases that are commonly used in the strategic planning process. The section that follows describes some of these terms to familiarize you with the language used in the development of strategies and your strategic plan.

STRATEGY

Strategy refers to a comprehensive and coordinated plan of action designed to achieve specific goals and objectives. This is most often articulated in a strategic plan.

STRATEGIC THINKING

Strategic thinking is the activity of analyzing complex situations, considering multiple perspectives, and generating innovative insights to address challenges and opportunities. This includes strategic planning as well as setting strategic goals and objectives for an organization. Strategic thinking focuses on developing an understanding of an organization's environment and includes identifying trends, patterns, and potential disruptions that could impact outcomes and organizational effectiveness.

STRATEGIC PLANNING

Strategic planning is a process to help operationalize strategic thinking by making organizational positioning and priorities explicit and then clearly communicating them to both internal and external organizational stakeholders.

ADAPTATIVE STRATEGY

Adaptive strategy focuses on flexibility, responsiveness, and continuous adjustment of tactics to accomplish organizational goals. In public health, adaptive strategy recognizes that the public health and health care landscape is dynamic and uncertain, and strategic thinking aims to equip the organization with the ability to adapt and evolve as circumstances change. Key characteristics of an adaptive strategy include flexibility, rapid decision-making, open communication, a learning focus, environmental scanning and scenario planning, and adaptable resource allocation.

STRATEGIC GOALS

A strategic goal is a high-level, long-term aim that is set to guide action and decision-making. Strategic goals are typically designed to advance an organization or entity toward a desired future state, and they provide a sense of direction and purpose. In some strategic plans a strategic goal is referred to as a strategic priority. Strategic goals often have a three- to five-year horizon. Sample public health agency goals may include the following:

- Have an agency workforce that is revitalized, sustainably supported, and effectively prepared to meet the current and future public health needs of our jurisdiction.
- Increase access to healthcare services for those living in underserved communities.
- Reduce the incidence of childhood obesity in our community.

Strategic goals may be further broken down into specific objectives and they may be assigned to specific departments or teams within an organization.

STRATEGIC OBJECTIVES

A strategic objective is a specific, measurable, and time-bound target that an organization sets to achieve its strategic goals. Strategic objectives are the building blocks or intermediate steps that, when achieved, contribute to attaining a strategic goal. It is best practice for strategic objectives to be SMART (specific, measurable, attainable or achievable, relevant, and have a specific time associated with their completion).[34] Some strategic planners use the term *strategies* instead of objectives to describe these steps or milestones in a strategic plan.

Using the sample public health goals described previously, sample strategic objectives could include the following:

- Strategic goal: Have an agency workforce that is revitalized, sustainably supported, and effectively prepared to meet the current and future needs of our jurisdiction.
  - Sample objective 1: Develop a comprehensive workforce development and sustainability plan that outlines the agency's workforce needs, identifies skill gaps, sets strategies for recruitment, training, and career advancement, and identifies funding for all positions by the end of year 1.
  - Sample objective 2: Enhance recruitment and retention strategies by implementing a new initiative to attract and retain top talent and reduce our agency's vacancy rate by 10% and by sustaining a 10% voluntary turnover rate by the end of year 2.
  - Sample objective 3: Strengthen agency succession planning by identifying and preparing potential successors for key leadership positions by the end of year 1.

- Strategic goal: Increase access to healthcare services for those living in underserved communities.
  - Sample objective 1: Develop and implement an outreach program to raise awareness about available healthcare services among underserved populations by end the of year 1.
  - Sample objective 2: Expand the number of healthcare facilities and clinics in underserved areas by 5% by the end of year 2.
  - Sample objective 3: Evaluate the feasibility of offering telemedicine and digital health solutions to reach individuals who face access challenges by the end of year 2.
- Strategic goal: Reduce the incidence of childhood obesity in the community
  - Sample objective 1: Implement evidence-based school nutrition and physical activity programs to promote healthy behaviors among children in all county schools by the end of year 2.
  - Objective 2: Collaborate with 80% of local pediatric and adolescent healthcare providers to screen and identify at risk children for early intervention and support by the summer of year 1.
  - Objective 3: Develop and implement an awareness campaign about the importance of healthy eating and physical activity for children and their families by the end of year 2.
  - Objective 4: Advocate at the local level for policy changes to improve the availability of healthy food options in schools and communities by end of year 1.

Objectives are often accompanied by tactical action plans to ensure that they are achieved within the desired timeframe.

TACTICS

Tactics are the ways in which objectives are achieved. Specific tactics will depend on the organization's strategic goals, objectives, and resources. For example, using one of the sample objectives, tactics may include the following:

- Strategic goal 1: Having an agency workforce that is revitalized, sustainably supported, and effectively prepared to meet the current and future needs of our jurisdiction.
  - Sample objective 1: Develop a comprehensive workforce development and sustainability plan that outlines the agency's workforce needs, identifies skill gaps, sets strategies for recruitment, training, and career advancement, and identifies funding for all positions by the end of year 1.
    - Tactics: Quarter 1, months 1–3
      - ◊ Establish a workforce development planning team of cross-functional agency leaders, HR professionals, and subject matter experts (month 1).
      - ◊ Conduct a workforce needs assessment (month 2).

  - ◊ Identify current and future workforce needs based on agency goals and objectives (months 1–3).
  - ◊ Engage with agency staff, stakeholders, and partners to gather input and insights on workforce development priorities (month 2).
- ■ Tactics: Quarter 2, months 4–6
  - ◊ Review and benchmark best practices (months 4–5).
  - ◊ Research and benchmark our agency against other public health agencies and organizations known for effective workforce development strategies (month 4).
  - ◊ Develop a draft Workforce Development Plan (WDP; month 5).
  - ◊ Outline strategies for recruitment, training, and career advancement (month 6).
  - ◊ Begin identifying potential funding sources for the workforce plan, including grants, partnerships, and internal budget allocations (month 6).
- ■ Tactics: Quarter 3, months 7–9
  - ◊ Finalize the WDP draft (month 7)
  - ◊ Circulate the WDP for internal review and feedback from stakeholders, including employees, managers, and agency leadership (month 8).
  - ◊ Refine the WDP based on feedback and insights obtained during the review process (month 9).
- ■ Tactics: Quarter 4, months 10–12
  - ◊ Finalize the WDP (month 10).
  - ◊ Create a detailed implementation roadmap that outlines tasks, responsibilities, and timelines for the coming years (month 11).
  - ◊ Secure initial funding or grants to support the implementation of key workforce development initiatives (months 11–12).
  - ◊ Develop a communication strategy to inform agency staff and stakeholders about the plan's objectives and implementation timelines (months 11–12).

The resources (financial, technological, and people) needed to accomplish each tactic and its associated tactics can be linked to each tactic to help clarify the effort needed to accomplish each task. Team workplans can also be developed for each tactic to help guide staff activities over specific periods of time.

OPERATIONAL PLAN

An operational plan is a document that outlines the day-to-day activities, processes, and resources required to implement the goals, objectives, and tactics set forth in a strategic plan. An operational plan provides a roadmap for how an organization will execute its strategic plan and translates high-level strategies into actionable tasks. It may also include metrics and key performance indicators, or those may be presented in a different strategic plan progress report or dashboard tool.

METRICS OR KEY PERFORMANCE INDICATORS

Metrics or key performance indicators are used to track and assess the performance and progress of an organization in achieving its strategic goals and objectives.

Appendix B: Resources for Further Study

There are numerous resources on systems thinking and strategic thinking in print and available online. Here are a few you may find helpful in your learning journey.

RESOURCES ON STRATEGIC PLANNING FOR PUBLIC HEALTH AGENCIES

These three resources provide overviews of the strategic planning process in public health agencies. All are currently available online with open access.

- Association of State and Territorial Health Officials (ASTHO). *Strategic Planning Guide: Guidance and Resources to Assist State and Territorial Health Agencies in Developing a Strategic Plan*. Accessed January 1, 2024. https://www.astho.org/topic/public-health-infrastructure/planning/strategic-planning-guide
- Kansas Health Institute. Strategic Planning in the Public Health Sector Handbook. April 2015. Accessed January 1, 2024. https://www.kansashealthmatters.org/content/sites/kansas/Training/strategic_plan_handbook_2015.pdf
- National Association of County and City Health Officials (NACCHO). Developing a local health department strategic plan: A how-to guide. Accessed January 1, 2024. https://www.naccho.org/uploads/downloadable-resources/Programs/Public-Health-Infrastructure/StrategicPlanningGuideFinal.pdf

WORKBOOKS AND HOW-TO GUIDES ON STRATEGIC PLANNING

These two books are tactical guides for conducting strategic planning in a variety of settings. I have used them both extensively in strategic planning workshops and retreats over the years.

- Barry B. *Strategic Planning Workbook for Nonprofit Organizations*. Fieldstone Alliance Publishing Center; 1997.
- Bryson JM, Alston FK. *Creating and Implementing Your Strategic Plan: A Workbook for Nonprofit Organizations*. Jossey-Bass; 1996.

BOOKS AND ARTICLES ON STRATEGY AND STRATEGIC THINKING

There are numerous resources on strategy and strategic thinking available in print and online journals, blog posts, books, and business websites on strategy and organizational behavior. The following list contains a few resources that I have found extremely valuable in my work on developing strategy and growing my strategic thinking competency. They build on the concepts described in this primer.

- Bryson JM. *Strategic Planning for Public and Nonprofit Organizations: A Guide to Strengthening and Sustaining Organizational Achievement*. Wiley; 2018.
- Drucker P, Collins JC, Kotler P, et al. *The Five Most Important Questions You Will Ever Ask About Your Organization*. Jossey-Bass; 2008.
- Harvard Business Review. *HBR's 10 Must Reads on Strategy*. Harvard Business Review Press; 2011.
- Horwath R. *Elevate: The Three Disciplines of Advanced Strategic Thinking*. Wiley; 2014.
- Horwath R. How to become a better strategic thinker: Three core behaviors to cultivate. *Harvard Business Review*. November 8, 2023. Accessed January 1, 2024. https://hbr.org/2023/11/how-to-become-a-better-strategic-thinker
- Lafley AG, Martin RL. *Playing to Win: How Strategy Really Works*. Harvard Business Review Press; 2014.
- Porter, ME. What is strategy? *Harvard Business Review*. 1996; 74(6):61–78. https://hbr.org/1996/11/what-is-strategy
- Steinberg B, Watkins MD. 10 ways to prove you are a strategic thinker. *Harvard Business Review*. October 31, 2023. Accessed January 1, 2024. https://hbr.org/2023/10/10-ways-to-prove-youre-a-strategic-thinker
- Zweifel T, Borey E. *Strategy in Action: Marrying Planning, People, and Performance*. iHorizon; 2013.

BOOKS AND ARTICLES ON SYSTEMS THINKING

These resources include a variety of current book chapters, articles, and entire volumes on systems thinking and the application of systems thinking to public health.

- Bender K. Systems thinking in public health. In: Helm-Murtagh SC, Erwin P, eds. *Leadership in Practice: Essentials for Public Health and Healthcare Leaders*. Springer Publishing; 2023:33–53.

- Branscomb J, Dills JE, Landers G, Minyard KJ, Hassmiller L. Systems thinking for public health professionals. In: Fraser MR, Castrucci CC, eds. *Building Strategic Skills for Better Health: A Primer for Public Health Professionals*. Oxford University Press; 2024:38–53.
- Cabrera D, Cabrera L. *Systems Thinking Made Simple: New Hope for Solving Wicked Problems*. Odyssean Press; 2015.
- Calancie L, Anderson S, Branscomb J, Apostolico AA, Lich KH. Using behavior over time graphs to spur systems thinking among public health practitioners. *Prev Chronic Dis*. 2018;15:170254. doi:10.5888/pcd15.170254
- Fraser MR, Castrucci BC, eds. *Building Strategic Skills for Better Health: A Primer for Public Health Professionals*. Oxford University Press; 2024.
- Ginter PM, Duncan J. Strategic thinking: rationale, process, and behaviors. In: Helm-Murtagh SC, Erwin P, eds. *Leadership in Practice: Essentials for Public Health and Healthcare Leaders*. Springer Publishing; 2023:55–76.
- Meadows DH. *Thinking in Systems: A Primer*. Chelsea Green Publishing; 2008.
- Rowitz L. *Public Health Leadership: Putting Principles into Action*. Jones and Bartlett Learning; 2014.
- Stroh DP. *Systems Thinking for Social Change: A Practical Guide to Solving Complex Problems, Avoiding Unintended Consequences, and Achieving Lasting Results*. Chelsea Green Publishing; 2015.
- Sweeney LB, Meadows D. *The Systems Thinking Playbook: Exercises to Stretch and Build Learning and Systems Thinking Capabilities*. Chelsea Green Publishing; 1995.
- Senge PM. *The Fifth Discipline: The Art and Practice of the Learning Organization*. Crown Business; 2006.
- Williams B, Hummelbrunner R. *Systems Concepts in Action*. Stanford University Press; 2009.

WEBSITES ON SYSTEMS THINKING

- POLARIS: This CDC website has several online trainings available on systems thinking topics including: Thinking in Systems Overview, An Introduction to Thinking in Systems, Thinking in Systems: Conversation Starters, and Thinking in Systems: Applying the Framework. (https://www.cdc.gov/policy/polaris/index.html)
- The Donella Meadows Project and The Academy for Systems Change: This website is dedicated to sharing the work of Donella Meadows and has several excellent resources and articles on systems thinking available for download. (https://donellameadows.org; https://donellameadows.org/systems-thinking-resources)

About the Author

Michael Fraser, PhD, MS, joined the College of American Pathologists as its Chief Executive Officer in March 2024 and was the chief executive officer of the Association of State and Territorial Health Officials (ASTHO) during the preparation of this manuscript. Under Fraser's leadership and in partnership with the ASTHO Board of Directors, ASTHO has received multiple awards including the 2022 Fries Prize for Improving Health on behalf of all state and territorial health agencies for their work to respond to COVID-19 and several Power of "A" Awards from the American Society of Association Executives for ASTHO's outstanding performance. Fraser has been featured in interviews with the *Washington Post, New York Times, Wall Street Journal, Politico, The Hill, CNN, Bloomberg, MSNBC, Governing*, and other national and regional media outlets. He is the author of over 40 peer-reviewed scientific publications and commentaries and contributed to several book projects including as co-author of *Vaccinating America: The Inside Story Behind the Race to Vaccinate America, Save Lives, and End a Pandemic*, and co-editor and author of *A Public Health Guide to Ending the Opioid Crisis* and *A Communications Playbook for Public Officials: How to Effectively Manage the Message, the Media, and Yourself.* He is also co-editor of *Building Strategic Skills for Better Health: A Primer for Public Health Professionals.* Fraser received his PhD and MA in sociology from the University of Massachusetts at Amherst and an MS in management with a concentration on management, strategy and leadership from the Eli Broad School of Management at Michigan State University. He received his BA in sociology from Oberlin College in 1991.

Index

Page numbers followed by *b* and *f* indicate boxes and figures respectively.

D

E

F

G

H

I

K

L

M

S

T

U

V

W